Using Whole Body **Vibration**
IN Physical Therapy AND Sport

Commissioning Editor: *Rita Demetriou-Swanwick*
Development Editor: *Veronika Watkins, Natalie Meylan*
Project Manager: *Nayagi Athmanathan/Anne Dickie*
Designer: *Stewart Larking*
Illustration Manager: *Bruce Hogarth*
Illustrator: *Robert Britton*

Using Whole Body **Vibration** IN **Physical Therapy** AND Sport

Clinical Practice and Treatment Exercises

Alfio Albasini

PT, PostGradManipTherap,
Private Practicioner
International Teacher, McConnell Institute,
Neurodynamic Solutions (NDS)
Member of CEC Otto Bock
Member of SUPSI and USI, Università della Svizzera Italiana

Martin Krause

Bachelor Applied Science (Physiotherapy),
Graduate Diploma Health Science (Exercise and Sport),
Master Applied Science (Manipulative Physiotherapy),
Certificate IV Workplace Assessment and Training
Graduate Certificate Health Science Education,
Back in Business Musculoskeletal & Sports Physiotherapy,
Pro Cure Physiotherapy Pty Ltd Australia.

Ingo Volker Rembitzki

Physical therapist, Certified MT and MLT,
Chairman of the Clinical Excellence Circle of Otto Bock Health Care Company,
Project manager Medical Affairs; Instructor WBV therapy.

FOREWORD BY
Martha R. Hinman, PT, EdD
Professor, Dept. of Physical Therapy,
Director, Transitional DPT Program,
Hardin-Simmons University.

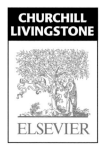

Edinburgh   London   New York   Oxford   Philadelphia   St Louis   Sydney   Toronto   2010

CHURCHILL
LIVINGSTONE
ELSEVIER

First published 2010, © Elsevier Limited. All rights reserved.

ISBN 978 0 7020 3173 1

British Library Cataloguing in Publication Data
A catalogue record for this book is available from the British Library

Library of Congress Cataloging in Publication Data
A catalog record for this book is available from the Library of
Congress

Notice
Knowledge and best practice in this field are constantly changing. As
new research and experience broaden our knowledge, changes in
practice, treatment and drug therapy may become necessary or
appropriate. Readers are advised to check the most current
information provided (i) on procedures featured or (ii) by the
manufacturer of each product to be administered, to verify the
recommended dose or formula, the method and duration of
administration, and contraindications. It is the responsibility of the
practitioner, relying on their own experience and knowledge of the
patient, to make diagnoses, to determine dosages and the best
treatment for each individual patient, and to take all appropriate
safety precautions. To the fullest extent of the law, neither the
Publisher nor the Authors assumes any liability for any injury and/or
damage to persons or property arising out of or related to any use of
the material contained in this book.

The Publisher

ELSEVIER your source for books,
journals and multimedia
in the health sciences
www.elsevierhealth.com

Working together to grow
libraries in developing countries
www.elsevier.com | www.bookaid.org | www.sabre.org

ELSEVIER BOOK AID
International Sabre Foundation

The
publisher's
policy is to use
**paper manufactured
from sustainable forests**

Printed in China

Contents

Foreward by Professor Martha R. Hinman

The influence of new technology on the practice of physical therapy and sports medicine continues to challenge our ability to scientifically test the efficacy of products designed to enhance physical performance. Whole body vibration (WBV) equipment is one example of this new technology. Although it is difficult to estimate the current number of companies that market WBV equipment, the number has grown exponentially in recent years; a Google™ search will produce close to 150,000 web sites, depending on the search terms used. Skeptics of WBV claim that this just another fitness fad, while other critics cite the 'unproven claims' made by WBV manufacturers who are hoping to cash in on consumer demands for new cures to old health care problems.

Over the past 5–10 years, I have received hundreds of phone calls and e-mails from individuals worldwide who are seeking health care advice on the benefits of WBV for conditions ranging from motor weaknesses to osteoporosis to autism. Unfortunately most health care professionals, like myself, are faced with more questions than answers when it comes to WBV exercise. Thus, these authors have helped to fill this information void by providing the first in-depth analysis and synthesis of the growing body of research on whole body vibration. They have coupled the results of numerous published studies with their own vast experience to provide an overview of the biomechanical and physiological effects of whole body vibration, as well as training guidelines to address a variety of physical impairments and functional goals. Whether your professional background is in sport science or rehabilitation, you will find evidence-based treatment parameters for improving muscle strength and power, soft tissue flexibility, balance and postural stability, bone density, peripheral circulation, and more. In chapters 5 and 6, the authors have also provided an illustrated, stepwise guide to help the novice practitioner utilize this new exercise modality in a safe and effective manner.

These authors, and the researchers whose work they have drawn from, have given us an excellent start. Like any initial work, this text is not necessarily an exhaustive review on the subject, but it does provide the scientific basis, clinical rationale, and treatment parameters needed to incorporate WBV into a physical therapy treatment plan or athletic training regimen with a reasonable assurance of success. And, hopefully, the outcomes experienced by these patients and athletes will be documented and added to the burgeoning body of knowledge that is needed for WBV to gain universal acceptance as a standard part of our clinical practice.

Martha R. Hinman, PT, EdD
Professor, Dept. of Physical Therapy
Director, Transitional DPT Program
Hardin-Simmons University
Abilene, TX 79698-6065
325-670-5828

Acknowledgements

I would like to commence by acknowledging my colleagues and coauthors, Ingo Rembitzki and Martin Krause. In particular, the latter has tirelessly given a major contribution to our book and without him this book would never have happened.

A special thanks is addressed to Salvatore Germano for his technical support during all the difficulties we had with our software and hardware.

I would like to thank Giuseppe Sarcinella, who created the photographs as well as the video.

I would like to acknowledge Federica Nobile for her contribution, as a volunteer, for spending several hours on the platform during the shooting in order to obtain the optimal angle for the photos.

Special thanks is extended to Natalie Meylan, Development Editor, for her great support whilst obtaining all the permissions we needed for this book and Rita Demetriou-Swanwick, Commissioning Editor, who helped me through the process of writing this book.

Lastly, the person who deserves the most gratitude of all is my wife, Astrid. She not only supported me during the entire period of this work, but she also took care of our two daughters, Aline and Aisha, during my absence due to international teaching and congress commitments. I will always be grateful to her because she allowed me the possibilities to achieve so many different steps during my career, always assisting me and protecting me and I hope that this book will give her some satisfaction as well.

Alfio Albasini

I would like to thank my co-authors and the publishers for their time and patience in developing this book. Furthermore, I'd like to express my deepest gratitude to all my teachers past and present who have imparted their wisdom and knowledge. The scientific advancement of Australian Musculoskeletal Physiotherapy is a telling tribute to these people. With the edition of this book I hope that I can also serve to stimulate and advance the art & craft of clinical practice through the Applied Sciences. Finally, I would like to dedicate this book to my parents Norbert & Sonja – who have always supported me, and my wife, Marianne and my son, Saxon who give me so much joy and happiness.

Martin Krause

I would like to express my gratitude to my friends Alfio Albasini and Martin Krause, my co-authors, for their good cooperation and excellence support. I would like to thank my family, my wife and my kids Rahel and Fabio Laurent for their understanding and support during the entire period of this work and all the professional colleagues and specialists who have helped me to become a specialist in this new field of whole body vibration training therapy over the last 9 years. I would also like to thank my patients for their patience and excellent cooperation during the practical work. My quite special gratitude goes to Prof. Felsenberg from whom I learned much more than just WBV through his work on bone material and muscle reactions.

Lastly, I would like to acknowledge Dr. Martin Runge, the Person who taught me the basics of WBV in the fields of geriatrics, muscle and bone physiologies.

I hope this book can contribute to the learning and understanding which is evolving in this interesting field of therapy.

Ingo Volker Rembitzki

Introduction

Alfio Albasini

Vibration training and vibration therapy, also known as whole body vibration (WBV), biomechanical stimulation (BMS), and biomechanical oscillation (BMO) date back to ancient Greece. Recently, vibration training has been reinvented as a new form of exercise that is becoming more frequently used to improve muscle strength, power and flexibility as well as coordination. Increasingly, WBV can be encountered in different wellness, fitness and rehabilitation centres as well as medical centres. Various professional sports clubs, such as AC Milan (soccer), Anaheim Mighty Ducks (ice hockey) and Chicago White Sox (baseball), are using WBV for their recovery and strengthening regimens in addition to their warm-up sessions. Individual professional athletes, including the legendary cyclist Lance Armstrong and Austrian skiing star Herman Maier, have incorporated vibration platform sessions into their training schedules.

Initially, vibration was used only for specific parts of the body (BMS). Later, a system with a counter movement (lateral or horizontal displacement) around a fulcrum was licensed in Germany, in 1996. Individuals using this tool could stand on their feet so that the whole body was stimulated with a sinusoidal vibration; hence the term whole body vibration was coined. This should not be confused with the vibration experienced in occupational injuries where the body passively vibrates over long periods of time. In the latter case, occupational vibration differs in its duration (e.g. heavy machinery driver) and also in the nature of its form, whereby sporadic movements are induced in the body, as in an air compression hammer, at a totally different frequency (>100 Hz) of vibration from that of WBV. The combination of duration and sporadic nature of movement appears, with the markedly higher frequency, to cause the deleterious effects. In contrast, WBV employs low-amplitude (<10 mm) and low-frequency (<65 Hz) mechanical stimulation of the human body for short durations (<30 min) to attain an effective and safe way to exercise musculoskeletal structures.

History

In 1880, Jean-Martin Charcot, a French neurologist, examined the surprising improvements in the condition of pilgrims suffering from Parkinson's disease. He surmised that such improvements were attributable to the vibration from the horse-drawn and railway carriages. Based on this idea he then developed a chair with a helmet that vibrated electrically. Between 1890 and 1910, Charcot's ideas were developed further by different therapists. G. Taylor (USA), G. Zander (Sweden), and J. H. Kellogg (USA) produced different kinds of vibration therapy for the arms and back. In 1960, Dr. Biermann, a West German, published the paper 'Influence of cycloid vibration massage on trunk flexion' in the *American Journal of Physical Medicine*.

In 1970, Professor Vladimir Nasarov developed a vibration training programme as an effective method for athletes. He observed an improvement in power and flexibility using Biermann's ideas in practical exercises. A short time later, this localized vibration training started to be used by the Russians in their space programme to prevent bone density changes in astronauts. They recognized that this new idea for exercise had the potential to provide suitable countermeasures for preventing bone and muscle loss for astronauts under microgravity conditions. WBV was later used to enhance the performance of Soviet athletes during their exercise training (Nasarov & Spivak 1985). These two authors were the first to highlight the association between strength and power development and whole-body or segment-focused vibration training. They assumed that repetitive eccentric vibration loads with small amplitudes would effectively enhance strength, because of a better synchronization of motor units.

Professor Nasarov was a Russian athletics coach who first applied vibration stimulation in sport. Basically, he wanted to help athletic performance based on the principle that by applying vibration to a distal muscle it would be transmitted to more proximal muscles. The special device he used generated vibration at a frequency of 23 Hz. Professor Nasarov found that the vibration produced an increase in the range of motion (ROM) of the involved joint, speculating that a shift in the pain threshold had occurred (Nasarov 1991 cited in Künnemeyer &

Schmidtbleicher 1997). He also hypothesized that vibration training, besides improving flexibility, would also improve blood flow.

The first study (Fig. 1.1) which combined weight training and vibration training was performed by Issurin et al (1994). These researchers found a 46% improvement after weight training with vibration (3 weeks, three times a week, 44-Hz frequency with amplitude of 3 mm, 30 m/s²). The same weight training without vibration had a progression of only 16%.

In a second study presented by Issurin and Tenenbaum (1999), 14 amateur and 14 elite athletes were subjected to vibratory stimulation during bilateral biceps curl exercises (Fig. 1.2) at a frequency of 44 Hz and with an oscillation of 3 mm peak to peak. They were also engaged in power exercises without vibration. The results in the elite athletes were an increase in explosive strength exertion for maximal and mean power of 10.4 and 10.2%, respectively, whereas in the amateurs the improvement was 7.9 to 10.7%.

In 1996, the first side-alternating vibration platform simulating the human gait was licensed in Germany. By 1998 vibration platforms with

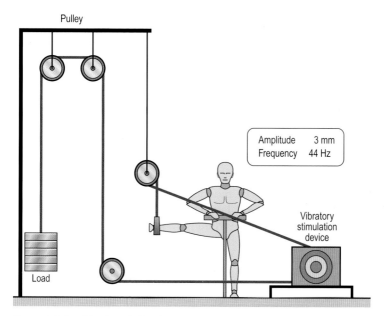

Figure 1.1 Combination of vibration training and weight training.

Reprinted from Issurin VB, Liebermann DG, Tenenbaum G (1994) Effect of vibratory stimulation training on maximal force and flexibility, Journal of Sports Sciences 12: 561–566, 1994, with permission from Taylor & Francis.

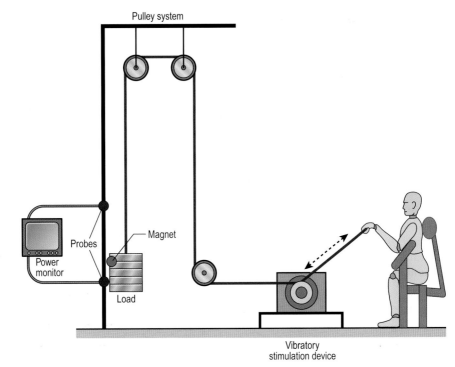

Figure 1.2 The bilateral biceps curl exercise and instrumentation.

Reprinted from Issurin VB, Tenenbaum G (1999) Acute and residual effects of vibratory stimulation on explosive strength in elite and amateur athletes. Journal of Sports Sciences 17: 177–182, with permission from Taylor & Francis.

various types of displacement were available on the market. Those oscillating vertically have a different frequency from those oscillating side to side. Exercise programmes incorporating WBV have been tested in the areas of sports muscle strength, muscle power and muscle length (Bosco et al 1999a, Delecluse et al 2003, Issurin & Tenenbaum 1999); in gerontology, proprioception and balance training (Bautmans et al 2005, Bogaerts et al 2007, Runge et al 2000), bone density (Felsenberg 2004, Gusi et al 2006, Rittweger & Felsenberg 2004, Rubin et al 2002) and the rehabilitation of various musculoskeletal impairments associated with disuse atrophy, muscle spasms and low back pain (Belavý et al 2008, Fontana et al 2005, Rittweger et al 2002); and in people suffering from the effects of stroke (Tihanyi et al 2007, van Nes et al 2004) and Parkinson's disease (Haas et al 2006).

Is vibration a natural stimulus?

During daily activity our body interacts with external forces. During walking and running our heel strikes the ground and absorbs this shock through pronation of the foot (McConnell 2002) and flexion of the knee (Perry 1992). These forces can also induce vibration and oscillations within the tissues of the body. Similarly, impacts related to sporting activity such as hitting the ball with a tennis racquet induce vibration. During, downhill mountain biking, vibrations are dissipated in the tissues through the arms. During downhill skiing, vibrations under the skis are captured by the body. Hence, through various structures such as soft tissues, bone, cartilage, synovial fluid, muscular activity and joint kinematics, the body not only dissipates the impact of the shocks, but also has a mechanism which regulates the transmission of these external forces (vibrations) into the tissue of the body (Cardinale & Wakeling 2005). It appears that the body is capable of tuning its muscle activity in order to reduce the vibrations that are passing through the soft tissue and which could have detrimental effects on it (Nigg 1997). Importantly, the amount of muscle activity required is related to the level of external vibration forces applied. A maximal activated muscle can dampen vibrations so that the oscillations within the tissues are diminished or eliminated (Wakeling et al 2002).

A 'concept of tissue homeostasis, the envelope of function', was proposed by Dye (1996), in order to explain anterior knee pain. This concept can be generalized to any musculoskeletal condition where the amount and frequency of loading is considered too large for the underlying structures. For example, while a weightlifter can normally lift over three times his body weight without any problems, a normal worker would not be able to do such a task and would probably become injured from such a huge effort. In such an instance, the normal worker would be outside his threshold, which could result in tissue breakdown (McConnell 2003). Dye (1996) described four factors pertinent to determining the size of the envelope of function: anatomical (involving morphology and biomechanical characteristics of tissue), kinematic (involving dynamic control of the joint), physiological (involving the mechanism of molecular and cellular homeostasis that determines the quality and rate of repair of the damaged tissues) and treatment (including the type of rehabilitation conducted by the therapist or the type of surgery that the patient has received).

Muscle can dampen external vibration and increase its activity in order to tolerate more vibration energy (Ettema & Huijing 1994). However, one must bear in mind that, according to Dye's theory, the body needs a certain time to adjust to the load, and therefore probably to vibration.

Definition

What is WBV, how can we define it?

WBV is a mechanical stimulus characterized by oscillatory motion delivered to the entire body from a platform. The devices currently available use two different systems: (a) a vertical vibration, meaning the whole plate oscillates uniformly up and down with only a vertical translation; and (b) reciprocating vertical displacements on the left and right side of a fulcrum, increasing the lateral accelerations. Biomechanical parameters, included in WBV training, are body position, amplitude, frequency, magnitude and duration.

The effects on WBV depend on the training parameters being used:

- amplitude–the extent of the oscillatory motion, peak-to-peak vertical displacement in millimetres;
- frequency–the number of impulses delivered per second (repetition rate of the cycles of oscillation), in hertz (Hz);
- magnitude–the acceleration of the movement, in g's (where 1 g is the acceleration due the Earth's gravitational field or 9.81 m/s^2); and
- duration–the total amount of time that a person spends on the platform, in seconds or minutes.

Considering the numerous combinations of variables possible, it is apparent that there are a wide variety of WBV platforms and training possibilities available. Furthermore, with the ability to differently position the body as well as using some external loads, such as rubber bands or weight, there are a lot of training possibilities.

Commercial devices that deliver WBV

There are different commercial devices delivering WBV: Galileo and Vibraflex platforms are manufactured by Novotec (Pforzheim, Germany) and distributed in the USA by Orthometrix Inc. (White Plains, NY); NEMES and NBS are manufactured by Nemesis (The Netherlands) and FitMedCorp. (Cleveland Heights, OH); Power Plate, Power Plate International (London, UK); and Pneu Vibe, manufactured by Pneumex (Sandpoint, ID).

Galileo

The platform works like a seesaw or teeterboard with an amplitude between 0 and 6 mm (equivalent to 0.12 mm peak to peak, medial to distal) and adjustable frequency, i.e. 5–30 Hz (oscillations per second). Basically, all the platforms from Galileo have nearly the same frequency and amplitude. The maximum is achieved by Galileo Sport, where amplitudes from 0 to 12.8 mm (peak to peak) and from 5 to 30 Hz are possible. Galileo Basis already has amplitude from 0 to 8 mm, and frequency between 12 and 27 Hz. The fast, side-alternating movement (side-alternating vibration training or side-alternating WBV) of the Galileo training platform elicits so-called 'stretch-reflexes' in the muscles, which cause muscle contractions and relaxation, from the legs up into the trunk and all the way up to the head (Ribot-Ciscar et al 1998, Rittweger et al 2002 cited in Cardinale & Bosco 2003). These reflexes are detached from the trainee's intentions and are controlled by the spinal cord. The number of stretch-reflexes per second is controlled via the adjustable training frequency. By choosing, for example, 25 Hz, there are 25 contraction cycles induced in each of the flexor and extensor muscles, which adds up to 1500 cycles per minute! This frequency corresponds with the time required for a single up–down movement to cause a natural stretch-reflex plus relaxation of the agonists and antagonists. The side-alternating up–down function of the Galileo platform simulates the human gait, which makes Galileo training a physiological training. This is the main characteristic which sets this platform apart from those which have purely an up–down movement.

Another characteristic which makes this platform quite different from others is the possibility of positioning the feet differently. The platform oscillates from the middle point, called zero (0) (the fulcrum is where obviously no oscillation takes place), to the largest point, called 4, where the displacement increases to 6 mm (10 mm). It is clear that the position of the foot, towards 0, or towards 4, will differently influence the entire body just by standing straight. Feet positioned more laterally have a different input because of the increasing lateral acceleration and amplitude.

Galileo Up-X Dumbell and Galileo TOP Dumbell

Galileo dumbbells (DB) are electric-powered devices which provide vibration to arms and shoulders and the upper spine. The handle, weighing 2.5 kg, centrally rotates, producing oscillatory movements to the body at different frequencies (0–30 Hz) with amplitude of 3 mm around a horizontal axis. Cochrane et al (2008) compared the effects of vibration on concentric activity with vibration utilizing a dumbbell with arm cranking. The result was enhanced peak power of concentric muscle maximal performance of 4.8%, which concurs with the results of Issurin and Tenenbaum (1999), where an 8% increase in peak power in male amateur athletes was seen. Similar results were achieved by Bosco et al (1999b), who reported that acute vibration increased unilateral bicep curl power output by 12% ($p < 0.001$) in national boxers. In fact the electromyogram (EMG) recorded in the biceps brachii of the experimental group showed a significant enhancement ($p < 0.001$) of the neural activity during the treatment period. The improvement of muscle performances induced by vibration training suggests that a neural adaptation has occurred in response to the vibration treatments. In this context, the duration of the stimulus seems to play an important role (Bosco 1985). However, the improvement of the mechanical power (P) noted after vibration training was not achieved by the EMG activity recorded in the biceps brachii, which was found to be rather low ($p < 0.01$). Issurin and Tenenbaum (1999) assessed the mechanical power of bilateral biceps curl exercise with a superimposed vibration of 44 Hz and an acceleration of about 30 m/s^2 transmitted through a two-arm handle. This was a special device which cannot really be compared to Galileo TOP but which gives a similar effect.

Galileo Delta Tilt Table

Galileo Delta Tilt Table is a system which can tilt the table and allow Galileo training even for walking/standing-disabled/-handicapped trainees. The amplitude here is 0–3.9 mm (0–7.8 mm peak to peak). The frequency varies from 12 to 27 Hz. There are tilt tables for adults as well as for children.

VibraFlex

The VibraFlex was developed by Orthometrix using the internationally patented Galileo vibration technology which is well known in the medical as well as in the sporting fields. VibraFlex is a device which functions in an oscillating pattern at a frequency between 5 and 30 Hz. The amplitude is 0–6.4 mm with a maximum displacement of 12.8 mm (peak to peak). This platform, compared with Galileo, has a preset frequency (6/12/18/26 Hz), preset time and preset training programme. VibraFlex has two handles laterally which can be used to attach straps in order to incorporate upper body exercises, increasing the intensity of the workout.

Mini VibraFlex, like Galileo, also has a handle and dumbbells, which are produced with the same technology. The frequency used is between 5 and 30 Hz, the amplitude is 2 mm, and the weight is 3.2 lb (1.45 kg).

NEMES and NBS

NEMES (*Neuro Mechanical Stimulation*) and NBS (NEMES Bosco System) are highly advanced computer-controlled systems of training based on Professor Carmelo Bosco's original ideas. Bosco was an Italian scientist involved in the world of sports physiology who invented the 'whole body vibration' method. The systems provide a vertical vibration between 30 and 50 Hz. At a frequency of 30 Hz, for example, each pulsation is given an acceleration of 54 m/s^2, which means that it is applied 30 times per second. The frequency and the acceleration at an amplitude of about ±4 mm results in a myotatic reflex or stretch-reflex. This reflex activity is also referred to as a 'tonic vibration reflex'. This means that the vibrated muscle has to work very hard, while the subject or player using the NEMES does nothing other than balance on the platform. The effect per pulsation is like that of the knee-jerk reflex. This muscle activity can be measured by EMG. For example, in one repetition of maximum effort, the muscle(s) involved are activated 100% voluntarily. However, according to NEMES, with vibration training the muscles work at 200–300%. This is an ideal way to train, especially when the muscle does not function properly, for example with weakened muscles in the elderly, or after injuries. This is what NEMES says, but one should be aware that some individuals, for example wakened by some neurological conditions, as Gillian Barre, or myasthenia gravis, or post-polio syndrome, will have increased suscepti- bility to neuromuscular fatigue and may not be the correct candidate for such a training protocol. NEMES has a powerful effect on muscle tissue, nerves, blood vessels, bones, fat tissue, cartilage, hormones and neu- rotransmitters. Further scientific-based explanations of WBV will be dis- cussed later in this book. The NBS Professional Model LX/LXB has a frequency between 20 and 55 Hz.

Arm Training (AT) NBS also has an arm training device similar to that of other companies.

Power Plate

Vibrating Platform was developed in 1999 by a Dutch Olympic Trainer, Guus van der Meer, who started to adapt acceleration training, first for elite athletes and then for people of all ages, weights and fitness levels. Power Plate has several devices; for example, AIRdaptive Power Plate pro5 can vibrate at a frequency between 25 and 50 Hz in a motion with a high and a low vertical displacement. The majority of Power Plate's devices have multiplanar motion with some devices having preset fre- quencies. No platform has a frequency below 25 Hz at the time of writing. Power Plate does not have dumbbells.

Pneu Vibe

Pneu Vibe has two models available, Pneu-Vibe Med and Pneu-Vibe Club. Both models have a frequency between 5 and 60 Hz and have only a verti- cal displacement. Pneu-Vibe Club is designed for use as a warm-up device, a strengthening device and a basic therapy tool. Pneu-Vibe Med has a larger platform that accommodates a wider range of rehabilitation exercises for both upper and lower body. There are a lot more devices which use the method of vertical displacement. These include Magic Vibe, Salveo, Fitplace, Fitvibe, Vibrofit and Bodyshaker.

Obviously, there are many companies on the market which are overstating the health benefits of WBV training. Each manufacturer considers itself to have the best WBV platform and that results are achieved in a very short time. So one can find statements such as 'it takes just two weeks to reach your optimal level of training just by standing passively on the platform.' Many companies market the results of WBV by expressing its ability to improve strength and muscle power, flexibility and mental stimulation as well as to decrease the effects of stress. Another important aspect to take into consideration is the quality of the platforms offered and the information given about the device. In fact some companies state a particular frequency which in reality is not correct and may be only half of what is written in the brochure. Often, cheap platforms have a maximal frequency of 15 Hz, and therefore it is not possible to achieve the different effects available at a greater range of frequencies (see Chapter 4 for a discussion of effects based on dosage and progression).

References

Bautmans I, Van Hees E, Lemper J-C et al (2005) The feasibility of whole body vibration in institutionalised elderly persons and its influence on muscle performance, balance and mobility: a randomised controlled trial. *BMC Geriatrics* 5:17.

Belavý DL, Hides JA, Wilson SJ et al (2008) Resistive simulated weight bearing exercise with whole body vibration reduces lumbar spine deconditioning in bed-rest. *Spine* 33(5):121–131.

Biermann W (1960) Influence of cycloid vibration massage on trunk flexion. *American Journal of Physical Medicine* 39:219–224.

Bogaerts A, Delecluse C, Claessens AL et al (2007) Impact of whole-body vibration training versus fitness training on muscle strength and muscle mass in older men: a 1-year randomized controlled trial. *Journals of Gerontology Series A Biological Sciences and Medical Sciences* 62(6):630–635.

Bosco C (1985) Adaptive responses of human skeletal muscle to simulated hypergravity condition. *Acta Physiologica Scandinavica* 124:507–513.

Bosco C, Colli R, Introini E et al (1999a) Adaptive responses of human skeletal muscle to vibration exposure. *Clinical Physiology* 19(2):183–187.

Bosco C, Cardinale M, Tsarpela O (1999b) Influence of vibration on mechanical power and electromyogram activity in human arm flexor muscles. *European Journal of Applied Physiology* 79:306–311.

Cardinale M, Bosco C (2003) The use of vibration as an exercise intervention. *Exercise and Sport Sciences Reviews* 31(1):3–7.

Cardinale M, Wakeling J (2005) Whole body vibration exercise: are vibrations good for you? *British Journal of Sports Medicine* 39:585–589.

Cochrane DJ, Stannard SR, Walmsely A et al (2008) The acute effect of vibration exercise on concentric muscular characteristic. *Journal of Science and Medicine in Sport* 11(6):527–534.

Delecluse C, Roelants M, Verschueren S (2003) Strength increase after whole-body vibration compared with resistance training. *Medicine and Science in Sports and Exercise* 35(6):1033–1041.

Dye S (1996) The knee as a biologic transmission with an envelope of function: a theory. *Clinical Orthopaedics and Related Research* (325): 10–18.

Ettema GJC, Huijing PA (1994) Frequency response of rat gastrocnemius medialis in small amplitude vibrations. *Journal of Biomechanics* 27:1015–1022.

Felsenberg D (2004) *Die Ergebnisse der Berliner BedRest-Studie*. Knochen and Muskel-Neue Welten. Charité Campus Benjamin Franklin, ZMK.

Fontana TL, Richardson CA, Stanton WR (2005) The effect of weightbearing exercise with low frequency, whole body vibration on lumbosacral proprioception: A pilot study on normal subjects. *Australian Journal of Physiotherapy* 51(4):259–263.

Gusi M, Raimundo A, Leal A (2006) Low frequency vibratory exercise reduces the risk of bone fracture more than walking: a randomized controlled trial. *BMC Musculoskeletal Disorders* 7:92.

Haas CT, Turbanski S, Kessler K et al (2006) The effects of random whole-body-vibration on motor symptoms in Parkinson's disease. *NeuroRehabilitacion* 21:29–36.

Issurin VB, Tenenbaum G (1999) Acute and residual effects of vibratory stimulation on explosive strength in elite and amateur athletes. *Journal of Sports Sciences* 17:177–182.

Issurin VB, Liebermann DG, Tenenbaum G (1994) Effect of vibratory stimulation training on maximal force and flexibility. *Journal of Sports Sciences* 12:561–566.

Künnemeyer J, Schmidtbleicher D (1997) Die neuromuskulaire stimulation. *RNS Leistungssport* 2:39–42.

McConnell J (2002) Course's Notes: The Vertebral Column.

McConnell J (2003) The use of taping for pain relief in the management of spinal pain. *Grieve's Modern Manual Therapy*, 3rd edn, 433–442, Churchill Living-Stone, Edinburgh.

Nasarov V, Spivak G (1985) Development of athlete's strength abilities by means of biomechanical stimulation method. *Theory and Practice of Physical Culture (Moscow)* 12:37–39.

Nigg BM (1997) Impact forces in running. *Current Opinion in Orthopedics* 8:43–47.

Perry J (1992) *Gait Analysis*. McGraw-Hill, New York.

Ribot-Ciscar E, Rossi-Durand C, Roll JP (1998) Muscle spindle activity following muscle and tendon vibration in man. *Neuroscience Letters* 258:147–150.

Rittweger J, Felsenberg D (2004) Resistive vibration exercise prevents bone loss during 8 weeks of strict bed rest in healthy male subjects: results from the Berlin Bed Rest (BBR) study. Presented at the *26th Annual Meeting of the American Society for Bone and Mineral Research*.

Rittweger J, Just K, Kautzsch K et al (2002) Treatment of chronic lower back pain with lumbar extension and whole-body vibration exercise: a randomized controlled trial. *Spine* 27:1829–1834.

Rubin C, Turner AS, Muller R et al (2002) Quantity and quality of trabecular bone in the femur are enhanced by a strongly anabolic, non invasive mechanical intervention. *Journal of Bone and Mineral Research* 17:349–357.

Runge M, Rehfeld G, Resnicek E (2000) Balance training and exercise in geriatric patients. *Journal of Musculoskeletal and Neuronal Interactions* 1(1):54–58.

Tihanyi TK, Horváth M, Fazekas G et al (2007) One session of whole body vibration increases voluntary muscle strength transiently in patients with stroke. *Clinical Rehabilitation* 21(9):782–793.

Torvinen S, Kannus P, Sievänen H et al (2002) Effect of four month vertical whole body vibration on performance and balance. *Medicine & Science in Sports & Exercise* 35(6):1523–1528.

van Nes IJ, Geurts AC, Hendricks HT et al (2004) Short-term effects of whole-body vibration on postural control in unilateral chronic stroke patients: preliminary evidence. *American Journal of Physical Medicine & Rehabilitation* 83(11):867–873.

Wakeling JM, Nigg BM, Rozitis AI (2002) Muscle activity in the lower extremity damps the soft-tissue vibrations which occur in response to pulsed and continuous vibrations. *Journal of Applied Physiology* 93:1093–1110.

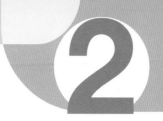

Biomechanics
Principles of WBV

Martin Krause and Alfio Albasini

The mechanism by which WBV works on the body is somewhat debatable. It has been shown that mechanical vibrations applied to the muscle belly or tendons are able to stimulate sensory receptors, mainly length-detecting muscle spindles (Hagbarth and Eklund 1966, Lance et al 1973). The primary endings of the muscle spindle (Ia afferent fibres), stimulated by the vibration of the muscle, facilitate the activation of the alpha-motoneurons causing reflex muscle contractions. This results in a tonic contraction of the muscle, referred to as the 'tonic vibration reflex', TVR, (Hagbarth and Eklund 1966, Lance et al 1973, Bishop 1974). Electromyogram data have revealed that this neuromuscular response, TVR, is mediated by monosynaptic and polysynaptic pathways (Bishop 1974) and results in increased motor unit activation (Burke and Shiller 1976). The effect of vibration is to elicit short fast changes in the length of the muscle-tendon complex. This input is detected as a 'type of sensory stiffness' through which reflex muscular activity will try to dampen vibratory waves (Figure 2.1).

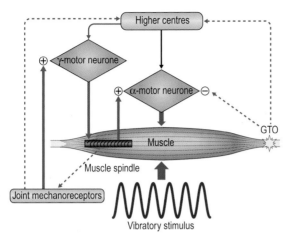

Figure 2.1 **Schematic diagram illustrating stiffness regulation during vibration stimulation.** The quick change in muscle length and the joint rotation caused by vibration trigger both α and γ motor neurons to fire to modulate muscle stiffness. Higher centers are also involved via a long loop.

Reprinted from Cardinale M, Bosco C (2003) The use of vibration as an exercise intervention. *Exercise and Sport Sciences Reviews* 31(1):3–7, with permission.

The effects of vibration depend on the properties of the muscle itself. The response of the TVR is influenced by the frequency of vibration, whether the muscle is relaxed or contracted, the level of pre-contraction of the muscle, the position of the body (static) or association with movement (in terms of whether a muscle is shortening or lengthening) as well as the combined effect of all the muscles surrounding the joint (Fontana et al 2005, Ribot-Ciscar et al 2002, 2003). The vibration is not only perceived by neuromuscular spindles, but also by the skin, the joints and secondary nerve endings (Ribot-Ciscar et al 1989).

In contrast to single muscle stimulation, the use of WBV involves applications to the entire body. The stimulation, which comes distally from the platform, has a long way to go before it arrives at the sensors. Along the way, the stimulus of the vibration will change and it is quite difficult to assess the quantity of this change. Roll et al (1980) applied WBV on seated subjects and concluded that vibration acts on the extero- and proprioceptive receptors rather than on the vestibular organs. Johansson et al (1990, 1991) revealed that vibration would result in increases in muscle stiffness and joint stability due a relationship between activation of joint mechanoreceptors and stimulation of the gamma efferents. In a standing position, vibration has an effect not only on muscles and tendons, but also on the joint structures, which means that an additional potent sensory motor effect through the proprioceptive joint mechanoreceptors occurs. This may also be an important factor in explaining the manner in which vibration may enhance proprioception.

Although TVR is the most proposed mechanism as to the effect of WBV on muscles, there is not a clear consensus in the literature (Luo et al 2005). The connection between WBV and the TVR has not been fully discussed and demonstrated in the literature (Nordlund and Thorstensson 2007) and therefore further mechanisms have been proposed in this book encapsulating the idea of stimulating future research into this relatively new field of therapeutic WBV.

To be able to understand the effects of WBV on human biological tissue it is important to understand the biomechanics of simple harmonic motion (SHM) of the machine. Inverse dynamics and tensegrity modelling in everyday functional activities aid in the understanding of the stabilizing mechanisms of human movement and how the body responds to rhythmic dynamic oscillations. Concepts of SHM and resonance frequencies, Young's modulus of elasticity and stiffness, and the development of torque, power, and work allow us to understand how kinetic and potential energy can be used as a training and rehabilitation stimulus. Through this application of biomechanics, the construct validity of WBV to functional movement, the hypertrophy of muscle and the maintenance of bone will become apparent.

The inverted pendulum and walking

Walking has been described as an 'inverted pendulum' whereby the body moves in the horizontal and vertical plane through a sinusoidal wave while the arms and legs are swinging like a 'normal pendulum'. This sinusoidal wave allows for the damping and acceleration required for efficient transfer of potential energy to kinetic energy and vice versa. The inverted pendulum is related to rocket or missile guidance systems where the thrust is actuated at the bottom of a tall vehicle. Similarly, in humans the thrust is activated through the feet into the body. The largest implementation of the inverted pendulum is in the technology of Segway, whereby shipping containers can be moved on cranes without the container oscillating. In fact, the inverted pendulum can be stabilized by oscillating the support rapidly up and down. If the oscillation is sufficiently strong (with respect to acceleration and amplitude) then the inverted pendulum can recover from perturbations 'in a strikingly counterintuitive manner'. If the driving point moves in simple harmonic motion, the pendulum's motion is described by the Mathieu equation.

Simple harmonic motion (SHM)

Understanding SHM allows the clinician to appreciate how WBV imparts vibration to the body and how variation of body position affects the rate of loading (acceleration) at the various body parts. Spring feathering systems occur when a body is hung elastically. Similar to a stretched rubber band the muscles gain potential energy when they are lengthened, which can be converted to kinetic energy and hence movement when they reverse direction. The efficiency of energy transfer will determine the velocity and acceleration of the movement gained. SHM simply is 'motion where the force acting on a body and thereby acceleration of the body is proportional to, and opposite in direction from the displacement from its equilibrium position' (i.e. $F = -kx$). WBV uses a range of frequencies up to 44 Hz to impart SHM to human tissue. The body reacts to this SHM in periodicities. Rubin et al (2003) used surgical pins in the L4 vertebrae to demonstrate that WBV frequencies in erect standing of less than 20 Hz imparted 100% transmissibility and therefore perfect resonance. Interestingly, at frequencies above 25 Hz this transmissibility decreased to approximately 80% at the hip and spine. Moreover, in relaxed stance transmissibility decreased to 60%, with 20° of knee flexion reducing this even further to 30%. This is clinically significant as it demonstrates that varying body position and joint angle will influence the site and rate of loading (acceleration) of the body part by WBV.

A general equation describing simple harmonic motion is

$$x(t) = A \cos(2\pi ft + \phi),$$

where x is the *displacement*, A is the *amplitude* of oscillation, f is the *frequency*, t is the elapsed time, and f is the phase of oscillation. If there is no displacement at time $t = 0$, the phase $\phi = \pi/2$. A motion with frequency f has a *period* $T = 1/f$.

Motor control: length, stiffness and potential

Interestingly these oscillatory concepts of physics were used in the 1930s by a Russian mathematician, Nikolai Bernstein (1967), to describe a solution to the problems of motor learning for the control of the degrees of freedom offered by the human body in the context of the environment in which it is interacting (Kelso et al 1980, Kugler et al 1980, Turvey et al 1978a,b, 1981). Specifically, these latter authors used the Bernstein perspective to account for the speed at which the movement control calculation was happening. They suggested that the CNS uses feed-forward mechanisms based on prior movement experiences to set the tone of the spinal cord reflexes required for synergistic muscle activity. Investigations into WBV and the effect of superimposed voluntary contractions revealed increased excitability of the α-motorneuronal pool as exhibited by an increase in the Hoffman reflex (Nishihira et al 2002). During functional activities such as walking, inverse dynamics and three-dimensional analysis have shown that the hip, knee and ankle are predominantly driven at angles close to 0° and 180°, or stabilized at angles close to 90°. Moreover, the three joints are never fully driven and the hip and knee are mainly stabilized during the stance phase of gait (Dumas & Cheze 2008). Harmonic motion as described by Hooke's law using a mass spring system analogy manages to account for the dynamics of a system of continuously altering control over 'stability' and its antithesis 'mobility'. The total muscle tone around the joints is represented by the spring (Fig. 2.2).

Although WBV represents a stimulus of exceedingly small magnitude and short duration, in terms of the repetition needed for motor learning,

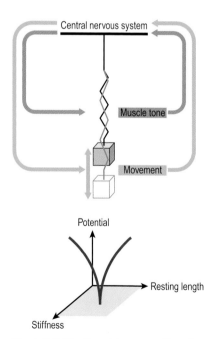

Figure 2.2 The Bernstein perspective of movement control using Hooke's law and mass spring oscillation.

Reprinted and adapted from Kugler PN, Kelso JAS, Turvey MT (1980) On the concept of coordinated structures as dissipative structures. I: Theoretical lines. In: Stelmach GE, Requin J (eds) *Tutorials in Motor Behavior* 3–45, North Holland, Amsterdam.

a 25-Hz stimulus for 1 min equals 60 s $\times$ 25 Hz = 1500 cycles, which may represent 1500 steps while walking or running. Sufficient cross-sectional area and muscle tone 'stiffness' together with proportional muscle length generates the potential of the system. 'Potential' may be expressed clinically as improvements in jumping, counter movement jumping, and enhanced scores in the items of the Quality Metric outcomes measure SF-36.

Clinically, neurological conditions affecting muscle tone, disuse atrophy conditions affecting muscle mass (sarcopenia) and overuse training conditions affecting muscle length will all have an impact on motor control and the body's ability to absorb and impart energy. WBV represents a novel training and rehabilitation form for the clinician as it can directly impart a stimulus to all three of these elements. Low-frequency vibration (<20 Hz) has been used to impart relaxation and change resting length (Haas et al 2006) or it can be used at higher frequencies (up to 44 Hz) to impart kinetic energy to the system, which increases the potential for movement through muscular recoil.

Because both velocity and acceleration can be derived from SHM equations they can be used to define the energy within a system. The amplitude of oscillation will depend upon the size (thickness, type of material and length) of the spring. Similarly, in the human body, muscle tone and body position will strongly influence the effect of energy capture and dissipation (Rubin et al 2003).

Stiffness

In terms of human biological tissue, these principles of physics can be applied using Young's modulus of elasticity whereby tensile stress and strain is used in conjunction with Hooke's law to define the elastic potential energy of the body part. During ambulation, as the heel hits the ground the muscles are stretched and gain kinetic energy, which is stored elastically and partially returned to the movement system as the muscle returns to its initial length.

Young's modulus, E, can be calculated by dividing the *tensile stress* by the *tensile strain*, which reflect the stiffness of the system:

$$E \equiv \frac{\text{tensile stress}}{\text{tensile strain}} = \frac{\sigma}{\varepsilon} = \frac{F/A_0}{\Delta L/L_0} = \frac{FL_0}{A_0 \Delta L}$$

where E is Young's modulus (modulus of elasticity), F is the force applied to the object, A_0 is the original cross-sectional area through which the force is applied, ΔL is the amount by which the length of the object changes, and L_0 is the original length of the object.

Resonance

Nikola Tesla (1856–1943) is considered to be the grand master of resonance. He experimented with both electrical and mechanical resonance. Some of his eccentric experiments caused mini-earthquakes in Manhattan. He managed to convince his friend Mark Twain to stand on a vibrating platform. Twain enjoyed it so much that he would not come off it when Tesla asked him to. However, a few minutes later Twain jumped off the platform and was seen heading to the toilet with diarrhoea.

A playground swing was one of Tesla's favourite examples of a resonant system. Each time the swing moves forward and then returns to its starting position it counts as one cycle. A stopwatch can be used to determine the length of time a swing needs to complete, say 20 cycles, dividing 20 cycles by the time gives the swing's frequency in cycles per second or hertz (Hz).

Since a swing is basically a pendulum it is possible to calculate its resonant or natural frequency using the pendulum equation as follows:

$$f = \frac{1}{2\pi}(g/L)^{0.5},$$

where g is gravity's constant (9.8 m/s^2 for Earth), and L is length.

Resonance and SHM are frequently used synonymously. If a structure begins to oscillate at its resonance frequency it is in danger of breaking if the amplitude of oscillations become too large. A classic example in the military is when soldiers break march when crossing a bridge.

Resonance can be seen with WBV and is determined by muscle tone, by body positioning and through co-contraction (Rubin et al 2003, Feltham et al 2006). Indeed, Mahieu et al (2006) used WBV to improve strength and posture control in young competitive skiers.

Wakeling et al (2002) examined the resonance and damping properties of soft tissue while standing on a vibrating platform. Fourier transforms were used to calculate the amplitude of acceleration as a function of frequency $a(f)$. The soft-tissue mass was considered a rigid mass for this analysis. For each given frequency f, the mean inertial power P required to oscillate the soft-tissue mass m was given by

$$P = \frac{ma^2}{4\sqrt{2\pi}f}$$

Hereby they stated that the total inertial power P'_t required for the oscillation in a particular direction is given by

$$P'_t = \frac{m}{4\sqrt{2\pi}} \int \frac{a^2}{f} \, df$$

Since soft-tissue oscillations occur in all three orthogonal directions, the total inertial power P_t required for vibration of all the soft tissues is given by the resultant power from all three directions (x, y, z) by

$$P_t = \sqrt{P_{t,x}'^2 + P_{t,y}'^2 + P_{t,z}'^2}$$

There was a time delay in response by the soft tissue of 150 ms, and this resulted in a decrease in the amplitude of the acceleration (Fig. 2.3).

Wakeling et al (2002) were able to demonstrate that elevated muscle activity and increased damping of vibration power occurred when the frequency input was close to natural frequency of each soft tissue.

Another investigation by Bazett-Jones et al (2008) examined the effects of WBV on acceleration by manipulating the variables of amplitude and frequency. Using an accelerometer they were able to show that 30 Hz at 2–4 mm = 2.16g, 40 Hz at 2–4 mm = 2.80g, 35 Hz at 4–6 mm = 4.87g and 50 Hz at 4–6 mm = 5.83g. They commented that less stiff people would require more neuromuscular activation to dampen the WBV stimulus.

Force exerted by stretched or compressed material

Young's modulus of a material can be used to calculate the force it exerts under a specific strain

$$F = \frac{EA_0 \Delta L}{L_0},$$

where F is the force exerted by the material when compressed or stretched by ΔL. From this formula Hooke's law can be derived, which describes the stiffness of an ideal spring:

$$F = \left(\frac{EA_0}{L_0} \right) \Delta L = kx,$$

where

$$k = \frac{EA_0}{L_0}$$

$$x = \Delta L.$$

E = Elasticity
A_0 = original cross sectional area
L_0 = original length
ΔL = change in length
F = Force

The relevance of compressed and tensile properties to humans becomes apparent when examining tensegrity modelling. Tensegrity views the

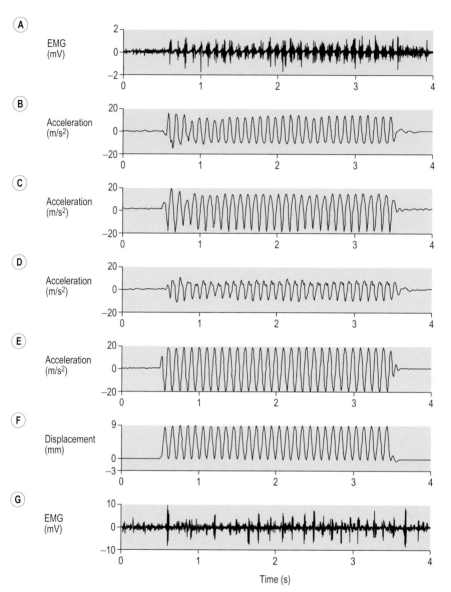

Figure 2.3 Electromyogram (EMG) trace from the medial gastrocnemius (A) and acceleration traces from the triceps surae (B–D) during one burst of continuous **vibrations.** Acceleration traces are shown for the direction normal to the skin surface (B), parallel to the tibia (C) and mediolateral (D). Platform acceleration is shown in (E), with the corresponding displacement in (F). The excitation frequency was 10 Hz, and the natural frequency for the triceps surae for this subject was 15 Hz. The equivalent EMG trace for the rectus femoris is shown in (G).

Reprinted from Wakeling JM, Nigg BM, Rozitis AI (2002) Muscle activity damps the soft tissue resonance that occurs in response to pulsed and continuous vibration. *Journal of Applied Physiology* 93:1093–1103, with permission from Penny Ripka.

musculoskeletal system as rigid bodies (bones and compressed fluid) situated within a mobile mass of muscle and soft tissue. As such the tension generated by muscles is countered by the wet and dry constituents of bone strength. Moreover, the pre-tension of muscles and other molecular cytoskeletal elements are thought to define the stability and movement capabilities of the human body. The understanding of tensegrity could fundamentally change the way we view the effect of WBV and will be discussed later in this chapter.

Elastic potential energy

As stated previously the length, cross-sectional area and pre-tension of the muscle will influence its ability to both absorb energy and to transfer this energy into movement.

The *elastic potential energy* stored is given by the integral of this expression with respect to L:

$$U_e = \int \frac{EA_0 \Delta L}{L_0} dL = \frac{EA_0}{L_0} \int \Delta L dL = \frac{EA_0 \Delta L^2}{2L_0},$$

where U_e is the elastic potential energy. The elastic potential energy per unit volume is given by:

$$\frac{U_e}{A_0 L_0} = \frac{E \Delta L^2}{2L_0^2} = \frac{1}{2} E \varepsilon^2,$$

where

$$\varepsilon = \frac{\Delta L}{L_0}$$

is the strain in the material. This formula can also be expressed as the integral of Hooke's law:

$$U_e = \int kx \, dx = \frac{1}{2} kx^2.$$

Given mass M attached to a spring/pendulum with amplitude A with acceleration a:

$$k = \frac{Ma}{A}$$

$$f = \frac{A}{t} = \frac{\lambda}{t}$$

$$T_s = T_p = \frac{1}{f} = \frac{t}{A} = 2\pi \sqrt{\frac{M}{k}} = 2\pi \sqrt{\frac{A}{g}} = 2\pi \sqrt{\frac{\ell}{g}}.$$

$$E_{tot} = \frac{kA^2}{2} = \frac{MaA}{2},$$

where k is the spring constant, M is the mass (usually in kilograms), a is the acceleration, A is the amplitude, λ is the wavelength, f is the frequency (usually in hertz), t is the time in seconds to complete one cycle, T_s or T_p is the period of the spring or pendulum, g is the acceleration due to gravity (on Earth at sea level: 9.81 m/s²), ℓ is the length of the pendulum, and E_{tot} is the total energy.

Therefore, where body weight is known and where the amplitude and acceleration of the WBV can be recorded, then the spring constant or stiffness of the system can be calculated. The use of accelerometers on various body parts during WBV may be a useful clinical method for determining resonance frequencies.

Hill model of viscoelasticity and motor control

In Fig. 2.4 it can be seen that WBV has the potential of affecting the viscoelastic elements of the tendons, fascia, and passive and active cytoskeletal

Hill model of viscoelasticity and motor control

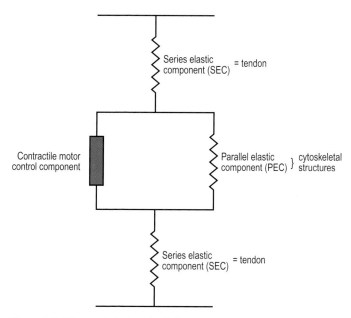

Figure 2.4 Hill model of viscoelasticity.
Reprinted from *Journal of Biomechanics* 14/6, Phillips and Petrofsky (1981), with permission from Elsevier.

structures. Additionally, the resting length of the contractile element and the rate and type of muscular contraction will influence the amount of energy absorbed and hence the recoil imparted when stretched. Unique cellular cytoskeletal myotubules will be discussed in terms of tensegrity later in this chapter.

Clinically, the Hill model is useful in terms of conceptualizing the appropriateness of different uses of WBV. When a muscle is too stiff it cannot elongate and absorb energy at the same rate as a flexible muscle. In such cases the rapid elongation of the muscle results in injury rather than elastic deformation and recoil. Depending upon the inherent morphology of the person being trained, a naturally hypermobile 'floppy' person may need power and stability training, whereas the naturally hypomobile 'stiff' person may need flexibility training.

Generation of torque and the conservation of momentum

In terms of human motion, principles of torque generation and the conservation of momentum have been applied to inverse dynamics calculations using torque and moments of inertia (Dumas & Cheze 2008, Silva & Ambrosio 2004, Zajac 2002). Inverse dynamics uses intersegmental models to represent mechanical behaviour of human limbs. The equations of inverse dynamics are derived from Newton's linear mechanics $\vec{F} = m\vec{a}$, and Euler's angular mechanics using equations involving the moment of inertia.

To conceptualize energy think about a person who weighs 100 kg. This weight represents a force of 1000 N. If a person steps up a 3-m step, 3000 J of energy is required. If this occurs in 3 s then $3000/3 = 1000$ J/s $= 1000$ W. In 10 s this represents 300 W.

The rotational kinetic energy of a rigid body can be expressed in terms of its moment of inertia:

$$T = \sum_{i=1}^{N} \frac{1}{2} m_i v_i^2 = \sum_{i=1}^{N} \frac{1}{2} m_i (\omega r_i)^2 = \frac{1}{2} \sum_{i=1}^{N} m_i r_i^2 \omega^2 = \frac{1}{2} I \omega^2,$$

where m is the mass of the accelerating body, v is the linear velocity, r is the radius, and ω represents angular velocity (in *radians* per second).

When a person jumps they apply torque to their joints through active concentric contraction and positive acceleration of muscles; on landing the lengthening and negative acceleration of eccentric muscles contraction allow the storage of potential energy for the next jump. Since a swinging platform represents both positive and negative acceleration then it also represents transformations from potential to kinetic energy. Moreover, the energy is directly proportional to the velocity and acceleration of the movement. Therefore, longer muscles have greater potential for acceleration, and thus the storage of potential energy and the subsequent release of this in the form of kinetic energy produces movement during the recoil.

WBV devices use stimulation frequencies between 5 and 44 Hz, with typical amplitude of 2–6.5 mm. Lifting the legs and variation of body position result in muscle lengthening, which affects the entire kinetic movement synergy. Furthermore, the reaction to muscle stretches results in reflexogenic stimulation of the entire neuromuscular system. As a consequence of high stimulation frequencies, the ensuing muscle tone represents the net stiffness of the system.

Inverse dynamics

The previous equations and discussions were used to highlight the nature of oscillatory movements in the human body using jumping, stepping and ambulation as examples. Additionally, there are numerous other examples of vibration encountered during daily activities. As such, WBV represents a unique stimulus to enhance the capacity of the body to capture potential energy and convert it into movement and hence function (Fig. 2.5).

Besides the stimulus produced by stretching, the back and forth movement results in action–reaction (Newton's third law) in agonist and antagonist muscles which ideally are used to optimize control of the neuromuscular system. Using a vibration platform allows the muscles the opportunity to learn their site-specific and timely sequential activation and deactivation across the spectrum of motor firing. This typical action occurs rapidly during bipedal activities such as walking and running in such a manner that the individual phases cannot be controlled by cortical activity. Instead, the CNS chooses starting points/postures/attitudes with a goal-directed orientation. Spinal cord reflexes, neuronal pre-tuning and the physical characteristics of muscles and their motor engrams from experiential learning are responsible for the motor control of localized movement. WBV constitutes a reflex element of the motor learning experience.

In the elderly population the functional movement capacity is determined by their ability to generate force, the feedback they receive in terms of proprioception, absence of pain, flexibility, cardiovascular factors and their ability to prevent falls. For example, the gluteal muscles need to

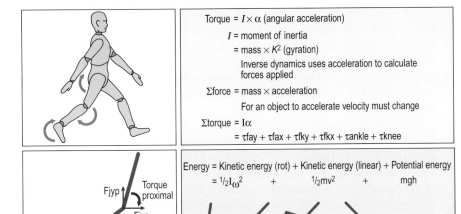

Torque = $I \times \alpha$ (angular acceleration)

    I = moment of inertia

        = mass $\times K^2$ (gyration)

          Inverse dynamics uses acceleration to calculate forces applied

Σforce = mass $\times$ acceleration

          For an object to accelerate velocity must change

Σtorque = $I\alpha$

          = τfay + τfax + τfky + τfkx + τankle + τknee

Energy = Kinetic energy (rot) + Kinetic energy (linear) + Potential energy

       = $\frac{1}{2}I\omega^2$ $\frac{1}{2}mv^2$ mgh

Increasing potential energy

Increasing kinetic energy

Fjyp, Torque proximal, Fjxp, Fjyd, Weight of segment, Torque distal, Fjxd

ω = angular velocity	g = gravity	f = force	p = proximal
v = linear velocity	h = height	d = distal	

Figure 2.5 The torque around joints using limb segments as levers to express the conservation of energy, using inverse dynamics, during walking and running. Any torque occurring at the ankle is transferred across segments through the 'energy straps' of the biarticular muscles.

Reprinted from Gait & Posture, 27/4, Riemer et al (2008), with permission from Elsevier.

generate in excess of 80% body weight (BW) in order to go from sitting to standing. Furthermore, the forward movement of the body generates a large lever for the gluteals across the hip and therefore requires flexibility. By requiring a torque the generation of momentum is required to overcome inertia, further suggesting the need for flexibility to generate the speed of contraction. WBV training certainly fulfills these requirements for a functional outcome such as improvements on the GUG test (Bautmans et al 2005, Bruyere et al n.d.). In standing enhanced stability in movement velocity, maximum point excursion and directional control were demonstrated to improve with WBV (Cheung et al 2007). Walking was also shown to improve in this population after WBV (Kawanabe et al 2007).

Eccentric exercise and plyometrics

Another parallel with exercise physiology and WBV are plyometric exercises whereby the muscle is forced to elongate and contract rapidly

(Fig. 2.6). The eccentric phase of contraction and the stored potential energy are supposed to enhance the concentric contraction and hence the ability to push or jump. A 'classic' test in sport is the counter movement jump (CMJ), which has been used by several researchers into WBV to validate efficacy. Anyone who has undertaken this form of training is conversant with the inherent risks of delay onset muscle soreness (DOMS) and its disincentive to novices to continue this form of training. WBV represents a novel and mild form of plyometric training which can be used as a warm-up to energize (>26 Hz) the muscles and as a cool-down to help relax (<20 Hz) the muscles. WBV can be used in the athletic population to both improve jumping performance (Torvinen et al 2002a,b) and prevent injuries. WBV has also been successfully used in postmenopausal women to improve their CMJ capacity (Roelants et al 2004).

The eccentric component to plyometric exercise causes more profound changes to the connective tissue of the muscle (broadening and streaming of Z bands). Investigations into eccentric exercise revealed pain 8 hours after initial exercises which was maximal 48 hours later (Newham et al 1983). These investigators found low-frequency fatigue 10 min after a 20-min period of stepping. Additionally, they demonstrated progressive increases in integrated electromyography (IEMG) during the exercise in the rectus femoris (160% increase) and vastus medialis (140% increase) in the eccentric contracting leg. Mechanical damage to the sarcoplasmic reticulum resulting in less calcium release for each excitatory action potential was suggested as the cause of the low-frequency fatigue. However, impaired force generation at a number of sites in the myofibrillar complex has been implicated (Green 1990). These include reduced binding sensitivity and capacity of troponin C for calcium, altered troponin–tropomysosin interaction in addition to impaired binding and force generation by actin and myosin. Indeed, the absence of any association between relaxation rates and calcium kinetics raises support for the notion of a rate-limiting process controlling the relaxation of fatigued muscles being located in the contractile proteins (Hill et al 2001). During fatigue the relaxation times can be prolonged by as much as 50%, thus resulting in increased force generation during submaximal stimulation due to tetanic fusion, despite a substantial fall in the maximum tetanic force (Bigland-Ritchie et al 1986).

The overall initial loss of force production seen may be due to desmin and titan damage (Lieber & Fridén 2002) (Fig. 2.7). Desmin acts as an extra-sarcomeric mechanical stabilizer between adjacent Z discs and the attachment to the costomere at the sarcolemma (Lieber et al 2002). The costomere complex contains talin, vinculin and dystrophin, which attach to the trans-sarcolemmal protein integrin and dystrophin-associated proteins. These proteins allow the lateral transmission of force from actin to

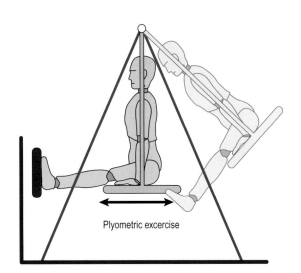

Plyometric excercise

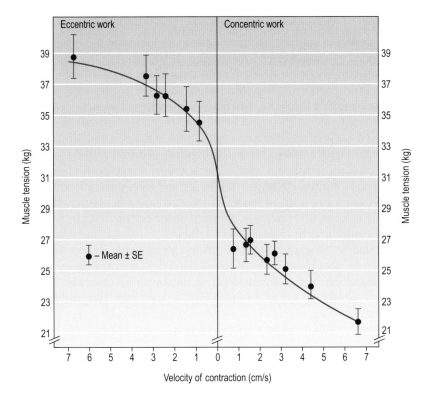

Figure 2.6 This graph demonstrate the inherent limitations in traditional forms of resistance training. It can be seen that as the load increases the velocity of contraction decreases, thus compromising power. Additionally, the loading angle and muscle resting length will strongly influence force generation. Such issues are largely ameliorated through eccentric plyometric-type exercise such as WBV.

Reprinted from Lichtwark GA, Wilson AM (2005) A modified Hill muscle model that predicts muscle power output and efficiency during sinusoidal length changes. *Journal of Experimental Biology* 208:2831–2843, with permission from The Company of Biologists Ltd.

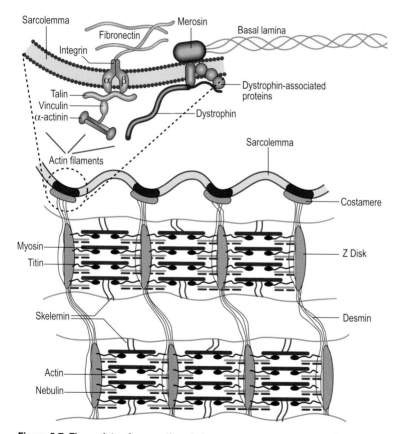

Figure 2.7 The variety of connections between structures provides a myriad of possible routes of force transmission and force transduction.

Reprinted with permission from Lieber RL, Shah S, Fridén J (2002) Cytoskeletal disruption after eccentric contraction-induced muscle injury. *Clinical Orthopaedics and Related Research* 403:90–99.

the basal lamina containing type IV collagen which is contiguous with the endomysium (Kovanen 2002). Desmin loss after eccentric exercise can occur within 5 min, possibly as a result of increased intracellular calcium leading to calpain activation and selective hydrolysis of the intermediate filament network (Lieber & Fridén 2002). This may result in the 'popping of sarcomeres' of different length, thereby potentially losing the myofilamentous overlap of actin and myosin (Lieber & Fridén 2002). Hence, reduced force production would be expected. Additionally, there is a release of matrix metalloproteinase (MMP), which may degrade the extramyocellular type IV collagen. However, this effect occurs many days after exercise (Koskinen et al 1996) and could even affect torque production 28 days after exercise (Lieber & Fridén 2002). This has significant implications in exercise training prescription whereby progressive loading improves functional capacity, whereas overloading reduces it.

Tensegrity

Although Young's modulus of elasticity provides a nice two-dimensional longitudinal explanation of stress and strain, muscle tissue forces also act transversely through cytoskeletal elements (Fig. 2.7) as well as at a three-dimensional cellular level. Tensegrity modelling has been used to describe stability and pliability of structures at a micro-(cellular) as well as macro-(skeletal) level. Tension-vectored forms provide discontinuous compression in a matrix of continuous tension (Fig. 2.8). Pre-tension is permanent and hence provides great strength relative to actual weight. Moreover, such a structure allows deformation without loss of integrity.

What is tensegrity?

Richard Buckminister Fuller defined tensegrity in his book *Synergetics*:

> The word 'tensegrity' is an invention: a contraction of 'tensional integrity'.
> Tensegrity describes a structural relationship principle in which structural
> shape is guaranteed by the finitely closed, comprehensively continuous,
> tensional behaviors of the system and not by the discontinuous and exclu-
> sively local compressional member behaviors.

Tensegrity is the exhibited strength that results 'when push and pull have a win–win relationship with each other.' Tension is continuous and compression discontinuous, such that continuous pull is balanced by equivalently discontinuous pushing forces. In the human body, pre-tension is provided by a matrix of connective tissue, whereas the bones and fluid provide the counterbalancing compression. In this model, rather than

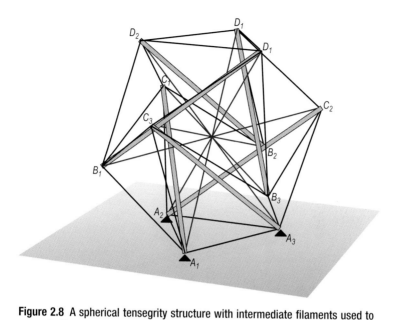

Figure 2.8 A spherical tensegrity structure with intermediate filaments used to generate the computational tensegrity model. The thin tendons represent microfilaments (black lines) and intermediate filaments (red lines); the thick grey struts indicate microtubules. Anchoring points to the substrate (blue) are indicated by the black triangles (A1, A2 and A3).

Reprinted from Sultan C, Stamenovic D, Ingber DE (2004) A computational tensegrity model predicts dynamic rheological behaviours in living cells. *Annals of Biomedical Engineering* 32(4):520–530, with permission from Springer.

viewing the body as being held together by bones, the reverse is postulated to be the case, whereby the soft tissues hold the bone spacers in place. Importantly, muscles and tendons and other musculoskeletal tissues adapt to the stresses applied at a molecular level which are orchestrated into a total body response. This occurs through the rearrangement of the molecular components that constitute the extracellular membrane (ECM) with interconnected cytoskeletal elements (Fig. 2.9).

Ingber (1997) stated that 'cells are hard wired to respond immediately to mechanical stresses transmitted over cell surface receptors that physically couple the cytoskeleton to extracellular matrix.' All living cells generate active tension in their cytoskeletal structure through an active actin–myosin filament, similar to that found in muscle. Therefore, all living cells have an internally equilibrated pre-stress. The intracellular cytoskeleton has binding molecules through focal adhesion complexes to the ECM as well as specialized junctional complexes at their lateral borders. Additionally, there are specialized cell–cell adhesion molecules. Transmembrane receptors that physically couple internal cytoskeletal

Cellular mechanochemistry

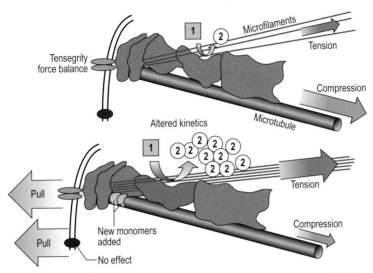

Figure 2.9 Contribution of cellular tensegrity to mechanochemical transduction.

Reprinted from Ingber DE (2003) Tensegrity II. How structural networks influence cellular information processing networks. *Journal of Cell Science* 116:1397–1408, with permission from *JCS Biologist*.

A schematic diagram of the complementary force balance between tensed microfilaments, compressed microtubules, and transmembrane integrin receptors and living cells. (1 → 2 is the chemical conversion of substrate 1 to substrate 2 which represents a change in kinetics.)

networks to external support structures provide specific molecular pathways for mechanical signal transfer across the cell surface.

Ingber (2003) postulated that the exposure of cells to physical distortion through their ECM is the requirement for developmental control, growth, differentiation, polarity, motility, contractility and programmed cell death (apoptosis) (Figs 2.10 and 2.11). Evidence for apoptosis comes from Huot et al (1998), who investigated the effects on actin dynamics of oxidative free radicals on stress proteins in endothelial cells. They demonstrated that the activation of the extracellular kinase (ERK) mitogen-activated protein (MAP) kinase pathway by H_2O_2 is essential for survival. Cells whose ERK was blocked displayed hallmarks of apoptosis, a thin F-actin ring with enhanced levels of HSP27 – an important heat shock protein. Enhanced localized concentration of HSP27 was postulated to be involved in modulating SAPK2-actin-dependent formation of membrane blebbing from its role in fibroblasts. Actin polymerization along with unconventional myosin pushes the membrane forward, whereas conventional myosin drives the retraction of the cytoplasm (Mitchison & Cramer 1996). The focal adhesions between the membrane and the extracellular matrix,

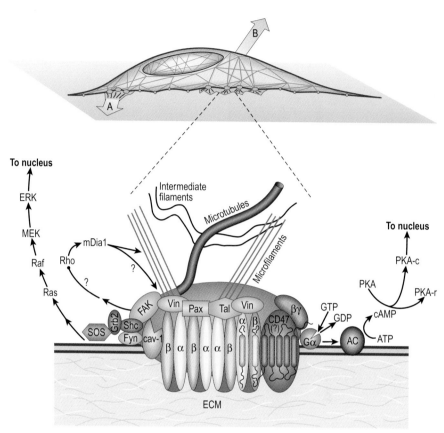

ECM = extra cellular matrix

α, β = dimeric integrin

Vin = Vinculin

Pax = Paxillin

Tal = Talin

FAK = Focal adhesion kinase

Gα = heterotrimeric G-proteins

ERK = extracellular signal-regulated protein kinase

cav-1 = caveolin-1

AC = adenylate cyclase

PKA = protein kinase A

ATP = adenosine triphosphate

CD47 = cluster of differentiation 47 (protein)

Figure 2.10 A schematic diagram of how forces applied via the ECM (A) or directly to the cell surface (B) travel to integrin-anchored focal adhesions through matrix attachments or cytoskeletal filaments, respectively.

Reprinted from Ingber DE (2003) Tensegrity II. How structural networks influence cellular information processing networks. *Journal of Cell Science* 116:1397–1408, with permission from *JCS Biologist*.

2 Biomechanics

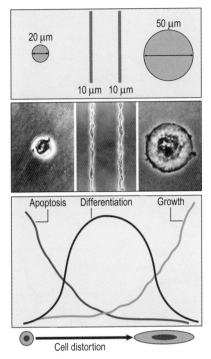

Figure 2.11 Cell distortion.
Reprinted from Ingber DE (2003) Tensegrity II. How structural networks influence cellular information processing networks. *Journal of Cell Science* 116:1397–1408, with permission from *JCS Biologist.*

and between the membrane and the cytoskeleton, are assembled after the recruitment of signalling molecules focal adhesion kinase (FAK) and paxilin with structural and membrane actin-anchoring proteins such as talin, vinculin, tensin and alpha-actinin. These proteins then provide a structural link allowing the anchorage of stress fibres to the membrane and to integrins. Huot et al (1998) argued that one of the pathophysiological consequences of weakness in this system is membrane blebbing, which could include narrowing of the vascular lumen, leading to increased vascular resistance and reduced blood perfusion. The effect of heat shock proteins (HSPs) on osteoporosis and sarcopenia will be discussed in the following chapter.

Ingber (2006) suggested that very physical perturbations can produce stress fractures of the cellular membrane, which alters the cytoplasmic biochemistry (Fig. 2.11). This frequently occurs with new exercise or increases in exercise loading. The degree of rupture produced by mechanical stress depends upon the dynamics of membrane resealing, which is controlled by depolymerization of cortical F-actin. Moreover, this regulatory process is dependent upon the pre-stress of the cytoskeleton. Ingber (2006) argued that the overall form of the cytoskeleton and the orientation of the cell relative to the load will influence the direction in which cells will grow. Isolated actin filament exhibits linear elastic properties, thereby obeying Hooke's law (Kojima et al 1994). Furthermore, the stiffness of these molecules remains constant over a wide range of tensile strains, thus supporting Sultan et al's (2004) assumption of the elastic linearity of tendon elements in the tensegrity model. Incredibly, actin, being a double helix, exhibits torsional rigidity and moments of inertia as it relates to Young's modulus of elasticity (Tsuda et al 1996). The unique nature of a sinusoidal oscillating stimulus such as WBV can be viewed as having the potential for the induction of mechanochemical conversion which is dependent upon the stresses being transferred over the spectrum of load-bearing interconnections of bone, muscle, fascia, ECMs, integrins, cell–cell junctions, cytoskeletal elements and nuclear scaffolds.

At a macrolevel, other researchers have used tensegrity modelling for robotics (Rieffel et al 2007) as well as aerospace research on passive and active damping of vibration (Chan et al 2004).

Additional explanations for the effects of stimuli such as WBV reside in the concepts of piezoelectric-crystal vibration and tensegrity modelling. In the realm of opto-mechanics these two concepts come together at material interfaces which are required for space flight. Geodesic domes and tensegrity structures are ridged, yet adaptable and dynamic. Most high-precision measurement instrumentation such as interferometers need to be ridged stable structures that do not drift or vibrate, but the alignments and phase shifting for measurements are usually controlled by piezoelectric transducers. In terms of the human body it may well be that piezoelectric crystal modelling is relevant to fluid dynamics and the hydroxyapatite calcium phosphate crystal complex of bone.

As an important mechanotransduction mechanism, it has been demonstrated that the response of bone cells to hydrostatic pressure and fluid shear stress is dependent on lipid rafts in plasma membrane cholesterol (Ferraro et al 2004, Yang & Rizzo 2006). Prostaglandin E2 Nitrous Oxide, data of flow-induced PGE2 and NO production demonstrate that the mechanical loading of bone is sensed by osteoblastic cells through fluid-mediated wall shear stress rather than by mechanical strain per se (Smalt et al 1997). Activation of fluid shear stress to osteoblasts causes the cadherin-associated junctional protein beta-catenin to translocate into the nucleus, where it activates gene transcription (Norvell et al 2004). Furthermore, depletion of plasma membrane cholesterol has been shown to dampen hydrostatic pressure and shear stress-induced mechanotransduction on osteoblast cultures (Ferraro et al 2004). Therefore, mechanical stimulation prevents osteocyte apoptosis through the activation of ERK

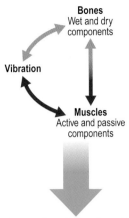

Bones
Wet and dry
components

Vibration

Muscles
Active and passive
components

Improved regulation of apoptosis
- Reduction in osteopenia
- Reduction in sarcopenia
- Improved immune function
- Improved lymphatics
- Improved blood flow
- Improved mobility and vitality

Figure 2.12 Summary of the biomechanical and clinical effects of vibration on muscle and bone.

via integrins and cytoskeletal and catalytic molecules such as Src kinase (Plotkin et al 2005). More recently, Skerry (2008) suggested that glutamate saturation of osteoblasts via glucocorticoid and/or kynurenine pathways was a mechanism whereby low-frequency WBV could maintain and even improve bone mass (Fig. 2.12). It is worth speculating that such mechanical strain may be induced by WBV both directly and/or indirectly through the hydrostatic elements within bone. The specific relevance to bone vibration frequency will be discussed in the following chapter.

Conclusion

Theories of motor learning based on principles of oscillatory bodies and an inverted pendulum were used to justify the construct validity of WBV. WBV represents potential anabolic stimuli at exceedingly low levels and duration of mechanical loading. Energy imparted into the body by WBV falls into existing theories on kinetic and potential energy, as well as simple harmonic motion, resonance frequencies and concepts of stiffness. Parallels can be drawn between plyometric resistance training and WBV.

Inverse dynamics explains the total kinetic chain impact of WBV. Similarly, tensegrity modelling was used to describe the stabilizing potential of WBV at a macro-level. Finally, at a microlevel, the tensegrity model suggests that stress proteins such as HSPs and cytoskeletal filaments help explain the potent anabolic effect of mechanical stimuli on soft tissue, blood vessels and bone.

References

Bautmans I, Van Hees E, Lemper J-L et al (2005) The feasibility of whole body vibration in institutionalised elderly persons and its influence on muscle performance, balance and mobility: a randomised controlled trial. *BMC Geriatrics* 5:17.

Bazett-Jones DM, Finch HW, Dugan El (2008) Comparing the effects of whole body vibration acceleration on counter-movement jump performance. *Journal of Sports Science and Medicine* 7:144–150.

Bernstein N (1967) *The Coordination and Regulation of movement.* Pergamon, New York appears in title of Fig. 2.2.

Bigland-Ritchie B, Bellemare F, Woods JJ (1986) Excitation frequencies and sites of fatigue. In: Jones NL, McCartney N, McComas AJ (eds) *Human Muscle Power* 197–213 Human Kinetics, Champaign, IL.

Bishop B (1974) Vibratory stimulation. Part 1. Neurophysiology of motor responses worked by vibratory stimulation. *Physical Therapy* 55(1):28–34.

Bruyere O, Wuidart M-A, di Palma E et al (n.d.) Controlled whole body vibrations to decrease risk and improve health related quality of life in elderly patients. Conference presentation, World Health Organization.

Burke D, Hagbarth K, Lofstedt L et al (1976). The responses of human muscle spindle endings to vibration during isometric contraction. *Journal of Physiology (London)* 261:695–711.

Burke D, Schiller HH (1976) Discharge pattern of single motor units in the tonic vibration reflex of human triceps surae. *J Neurol Neurosurg Psychiatry* 39:729–741.

Chan WL, Arbelaez D, Bossens F et al (2004) Active vibration control of a three-stage tensegrity structure. Presented at *SPIE 11th Annual International Symposium on Smart Structures and Materials.* [online]. Available at URL:http://maeweb.ucsd.edu/~skelton/publications/waileung_vibration_spie2004.pdf

Cheung WH, Mok HW, Qin L et al (2007) High-frequency whole-body vibration improves balancing ability in elderly women. *Archives of Physical Medicine and Rehabilitation* 88(7):852–857.

Dumas R, Cheze L (2008) Hip and knee joints are stabilized more than driven during the stance phase of gait. An analysis of the 3D angle between joint moment and joint angular velocity. *Gait and Posture* 28(2):243–250.

Feltham MG, van Deen JH, Coppieters MW et al (2006) Changes in joint stability with muscle contraction measured from transmission of mechanical vibration. *Journal of Biomechanics* 39:2850–2856.

Ferraro JT, Daneshmand M, Bizios R et al (2004) Depletion of plasma membrane cholesterol dampens hydrostatic pressure and shear stress-induced mechano-transduction pathways in osteoblast cultures. *American Journal of Physiology* 286:831–839.

Fontana TL, Richardson CA, Stanton WR (2005) The effect of weightbearing exercise with low frequency, whole body vibration on lumbosacral proprioception: A pilot study on normal subjects. *Australian Journal of Physiotherapy* 51:259–263.

Green HJ (1990) Manifestations and sites of neuromuscular fatigue. In: Taylor AW, Green HJ, Ianuzzo D et al (eds) *Biochemistry of Exercise*, 13–25. Human Kinetics, Champaign, IL.

Haas CT, Turbanski S, Kessler K et al (2006) The effects of random whole-body-vibration on motor symptoms in Parkinson's disease. *NeuroRehabilitation* 21:29–36.

Hagbarth KE, Eklund G (1966) Tonic vibration reflexes (TVR) in spasticity. *Brain Res* 2:201–203.

Hill CA, Thompson MW, Ruell PA et al (2001) Sarcoplasmic reticulum function and muscle contractile character following fatiguing exercise in humans. *Journal of Physiology* 531(3):871–878.

Huot J, Houle F, Rousseau S et al (1998) SAPK2/p38-dependent F-actin reorganization regulates early membrane blebbing during stress-induced apoptosis. *Journal of Cell Biology* 143:1361–1373.

Ingber DE (1997) Tensegrity: The architectural basis of cellular mechanotransduction. *Annual Review of Physiology* 59:575–599.

Ingber DE (2003) Tensegrity II. How structural networks influence cellular information processing networks. *Journal of Cell Science* 116:1397–1408.

Ingber DE (2006) Cellular mechanotransduction: putting all the pieces together again. *FASB Journal* 20:811–827.

Johansson H, Sjolander P, Sojka P (1990) Activity in receptor afferents from the anterior cruciate ligament evokes reflex effects on fusimotor neurones. *Neuroscience Research* 8:54–59.

Johansson H, Sjolander P, Sojka P (1991) A sensory role for the cruciate ligaments. *Clinical Orthopaedics and Related Research* 268: 161–178.

Kawanabe K, Kawashima A, Sashimoto I et al (2007) Effect of whole-body vibration exercise and muscle strengthening on walking ability in the elderly. *Keio Journal of Medicine* 56(1):28–33.

Kelso JAS, Holt KG, Kuglar PN et al (1980) On the concept of coordinated structures as dissipative structures. II: Empirical lines of convergency. In: Stelmach GE, Requin J (eds) *Tutorials in Motor Behavior*, 49–70. North Holland, Amsterdam.

Kojima H, Ishijima A, Yanagida T (1994) Direct measurement of stiffness of single actin filaments with and without tropomyosin by in vitro nanomanipulation. *Proceedings of the National Academy of Sciences of the United States of America* 91:12962–12966.

Koskinen S, Kovanen V, Komulainen J (1996) Type IV collagen MMP-2 and TIMP-2 mRNA levels in skeletal muscle subjected to forced eccentric contractions. *Medicine and Science in Sports and Exercise* 28:153.

Kovanen V (2002) Intramuscular extracellular matrix: complex environment of muscle cells. *Exercise and Sport Sciences Reviews* 30:20–25.

Kugler PN, Kelso JAS, Turvey MT (1980) On the concept of coordinated structures as dissipative structures. I Theoretical lines. In: Stelmach GE, Requin J (eds) *Tutorials in Motor Behavior* 3–45. North Holland, Amsterdam.

Lance JW, Burke D, Andrews CJ (1973) The reflex effects of muscle vibration. In: Desmedt JE (ed), *New Developments in Electromyography and Clinical Neurophysiology*, 444–462. Karger, Basel.

Lieber RL, Fridén J (2002) Mechanisms of muscle injury gleaned from animal models. *American Journal of Physical Medicine and Rehabilitation* 81(11):70–79.

Lieber RL, Shah S, Fridén J (2002) Cytoskeletal disruption after eccentric contraction-induced muscle injury. *Clinical Orthopaedics and Related Research* 403:90–99.

Luo J, McNamara B, Moran K (2005) The use of vibration training to enhance muscle strength and power. *Sports Medicine* 35:23–41.

Mahieu NN, Witvrouw E, Van de Voorde D et al (2006) Improving strength and postural control in young skiers: whole-body vibration versus equivalent resistance training. *Journal of Athletic Training* 41(3):286–293.

Mitchison TJ, Cramer LP (1996) Actin-based cell motility and cell locomotion. *Cell* 84:371–379.

Newham DJ, Mills KR, Quigley BM et al (1983) Pain and fatigue after concentric and eccentric muscle contractions. *Clinical Science* 64:55–62.

Nishihira Y, Iwasaki T, Hatta T et al (2002) Effect of whole body vibration stimulus and voluntary contraction on motoneuron pool. *Advances in Exercise and Sports Physiology* 8(4):83–86.

Nordlund MM, Thorstensson A (2007) Strength training effects of whole-body vibration? *Scandinavian Journal of Medicine and Science in Sports* 17:12–17.

Norvell S, Alvarez M, Bidwell J et al (2004) Fluid shear stress induces β-catenin signaling in osteoblasts. *Calcified Tissue International* 75(5):396–404.

Phillips CA, Petrfsky JS (1981) The passive elastic force velocity relationship of cat skeletal muscle: Influence upon the maximal contractile element velocity. *J Biomechanics* 14, Pergamon Press.

Plotkin LI, Mathov I, Aguire JI et al (2005) Mechanical stimulation prevents osteocyte apoptosis: requirement of integrins Src kinases and ERKs. *American Journal Physiology Cell Physiology*: 289:633–643.

Ribot-Ciscar E, Bergenheim M, Roll JP (2002) The preferred sensory direction of muscle spindle primary endings influences the velocity coding of two-dimensional limb movements in humans. *Experimental Brain Research* 145:429–436.

Ribot-Ciscar E, Bergenheim M, Albert F et al (2003) Proprioceptive population coding of limb position in humans. *Experimental Brain Research* 149:512–519.

Ribot-Ciscar E, Vedel JP, Roll JP (1989) Vibration sensitivity of slowly and rapidly adapting cutaneous mechanoreceptors in the human foot and leg. *Neurosci Lett* Sep 25;104(1-2):130–135.

Rieffel J, Stuk RJ, Valero-Cuevas FJ et al (2007) Locomotion of a tensegrity robot via dynamically coupled modules. *Proceedings of the International Conference on Morphological Computation, Venice, Italy, March 2007.* [online]. Available at URL:http://ccsl.mae.cornell.edu/papers/MC07_Rieffel.pdf

Riemer R, Hsiao-Wecksler ET, Zhang X (2008) Uncertainties in inverse dynamics solutions: a comprehensive analysis and an application to gait. *Gait & Posture* 27:578–588.

Roelants M, Delecluse C, Verschueren SM (2004) Whole-body-vibration training increases knee-extension strength and speed of movement in older women. *Journal of the American Geriatric Society* 52:901–908.

Roll JP, Martin B, Gauthier GM et al (1980) Effects of whole body vibration on spinal reflexes in man. *Aviation Space and Environmental Medicine* 51(11):1227–1233.

Rubin C, Pope M, Fritton JC et al (2003) Transmissibility of 15Hz to 35Hz vibrations to the human hip and lumbar spine: determining the physiological feasibility of delivering low-level anabolic mechanical stimuli to skeletal regions at greatest risk of fracture because of osteoporosis. *Spine* 28(23):2621–2627.

Silva MPT, Ambrosio JAC (2004) Sensitivity of the results produced by the inverse dynamic analysis of a human stride to perturbed input data. *Gait and Posture* 19:35–49.

Skerry TM (2008) The role of glutamate in the regulation of bone mass and architecture. *Journal of Musculoskeletal and Neuronal Interactions* 8(2):166–173.

Smalt R, Mitchell FT, Howard RL et al (1997) Induction of NO and prostaglandin E2 in osteoblasts by wall-shear stress but not mechanical strain. *American Journal of Physiology* 273:E751–E758.

Sultan C, Stamenovic D, Ingber DE (2004) A computational tensegrity model predicts dynamic rheological behaviours in living cells. *Annals of Biomedical Engineering* 32(4):520–530.

Torvinen S, Kannus P, Sievänen H et al (2002a) Effect of a vibration exposure on muscular performance and body balance. Randomized cross-over study. *Clinical Physiology and Functional Imaging* 22:145–152.

Torvinen S, Kannus P, Sievänen H et al (2002b) Effect of four-month vertical whole body vibration on performance and balance. *Medicine and Science in Sports and Exercise* 34(9):1523–1528.

Tsuda Y, Yasutake H, Ishijima A et al (1996) Torsional rigidity of single actin filaments and actin-actin bond breaking force under torsion measured directly by *in vitro* micromanipulation. *Proceedings of the National Academy of Sciences of the United States of America* 93:12937–12942.

Turvey MT, Fitch HL, Tuller B (1978a) Part V: Degrees of freedom co-ordinative structure s and tuning. In: Kelso JAS (ed.) *Human Motor Behavior: An Introduction.* Erlbaum, Hillsdale, NJ.

Turvey MT, Shaw RE, Mace WM (1978b) Issues in the theory of action: Degrees of freedom co-ordinative structures and coalitions. In: Requin J (ed.) *Attention and Performance*, vol VII, 557–595. Erlbaum, Hillsdale, NJ.

Turvey MT, Shaw RE, Reed ES et al (1981) Ecological laws for perceiving and acting: a reply to Fodor and Pylyshyn. *Cognition* 9:237–304.

Wakeling JM, Nigg BM, Rozitis AI (2002) Muscle activity damps the soft tissue resonance that occurs in response to pulsed and continuous vibration. *Journal of Applied Physiology* 93:1093–1103.

Yang B, Oo TN, Rizzo V (2006) Lipid rafts mediate H2O2 prosurvival effects in cultured endothelial cells. *FASEB Journal* 20:E688–E697.

Zajac FE (2002) Understanding muscle coordination of the human leg with dynamical simulations. *Journal of Biomechanics* 35:1011–1018.

Theoretical considerations in the clinical application of WBV to sarcopenia, osteoporosis and metabolic syndrome

Martin Krause

Whole body vibration (WBV) has been advocated as a training regimen for improving power in athletes and functional sit to stand, ambulatory, reaching and balancing capacity in the elderly. WBV has also been advocated as a therapeutic tool for improving several conditions including osteoporosis and sarcopenia. Although WBV is becoming more frequently used in gyms and among athletes, the effects on the musculoskeletal system have been reported most significantly in the older population and in those who could be considered as deconditioned or vulnerable, such as people undergoing prolonged bed rest or space flight. Because of the relatively recent development of WBV, some of the research supporting WBV is tenuous at best. Hence, this chapter will explore some of the theoretical possibilities and sites of action of WBV in diseases such as osteoporosis, sarcopenia and metabolic syndrome.

The majority of the literature examines the effect of WBV on muscle function. As stipulated previously, strengthening regimens using WBV have proposed that the mechanism acts purely on neurophysiological reflex mechanisms induced in the muscles, skin and joint receptors. Additional to these mechanisms, theories of tensegrity (Ingber 2006, Sultan et al 2004) suggests that direct mechanotransduction of vibration to 'cell–cell adhesion molecules' and unconventional myosin motors at a cellular cytoskeletal level are also likely to have a significant impact on the pre-stress and hence health of muscular tissue through the additional influx of mechanical kinetic and potential energy which the WBV imparts. Furthermore, theories from tensegrity may have an important bearing on explaining the effect of WBV on trabecular bone function.

Muscle function is commonly associated with the movement needed to participate in activities of daily living, including lifting and ambulation. These activities will have varying effects on metabolic function depending upon the degree of loading which determines the amount of stress perceived by the system. The degree to which the system can counter this load is the 'strain'. Primarily due to suboptimal muscle function, serious issues of morbidity with far-reaching economic consequences have occurred in recent decades from the increasingly sedentary nature of occupational endeavours, the passivity of leisure activities and the automation of transport. Metabolic syndrome alone will cost Western society trillions of dollars. Therefore, the optimization of muscle function should be a primary concern for many healthcare organizations, since strategies to reverse or prevent muscle atrophy are considered to address many of the comorbidity factors of diabetes, osteoporosis, cardiovascular disease and impaired immune function.

Sarcopenia

The loss of muscle mass commencing in the fourth decade of life is termed sarcopenia (Morley et al 2001). This has significant consequences on morbidity and vitality as skeletal muscle contains 50–75% of the human body's proteins and represents a store of energy and nitrogen which become a vital supply of fuel for the immune system, as well as a substrate for wound healing during malnutrition, injury and disease (Rasmussen & Phillips 2003). Lean muscle mass accounts for 90% of the cross-sectional area in active young men, but only 30% of that area in frail older women (Rosenberg & Roubenoff 1995). The prevalence of clinically significant sarcopenia is estimated to range from 8.8% in 'young old' women to 17.5% in 'old old' men (Morley et al 2001). Sarcopenia has far-reaching consequences for people's health including:

- immobility;
- impaired immune function;
- impaired bone structure;
- increased morbidity due to increased incidence/risk of falls;
- metabolic syndrome (diabetes, high blood pressure, hyperlipidaemia, heart disease and obesity); and
- low back pain.

Muscle atrophy is the first step along a cascade of events leading to sarcopenia. Whereas muscle atrophy is reversible, sarcopenia is considered by most people as non reversible. In turn sarcopenia leads to reduced mechanical loading of bones which generates osteopenia while body fat content is increased through the consequential reduction in basal metabolic rate (BMR). Since muscle mass is considered a 'sink' for insulin, the consequences of reduced BMR and increased fat content are magnified with the addition of insulin-resistant diabetes. Ideally, we maintain our muscle mass throughout life as most people believe that, once we lose it, it is gone for ever.

WBV and muscle function

WBV has been used successfully to reduce paraspinal muscle atrophy during 8 weeks of bed rest (Belavý et al 2008). Significant improvements in fat-free mass and a 24.4% improvement in knee extension strength was demonstrated after 24 weeks of three times per week of WBV (Roelants et al 2004b). In another investigation, using a population of postmenopausal women, these authors demonstrated improved knee extensor muscle strength (16%) and improvements in counter movement jump by 2.8% after 12 weeks of WBV training (Roelants et al 2004a). Enhanced stability in movement velocity, maximum point excursion and directional control was shown with 20Hz, 3 mins/day, 3 days/week of WBV for 3 months in older women (Cheung et al 2007). The results of a 6-week training programme of WBV with 42 elderly nursing home residents were presented to the World Health Organization; seven items of the SF-36 improved, which included physical function (143%), pain (41%), vitality (60%) and general health (23%). Also, improvements in the quality of walking (57%), equilibrium (77%) and, get up and go, (GUG) 39% were shown (Bruyere et al n.d.). However, a subsequent publication by the same authors demonstrated much less significant results (Bruyere et al 2005). Moreover, similar to an investigation by Bautmans et al (2005) (see Table 3.1), the standard deviations suggest that there were large improvements in some people and not in others. If this is the case, then individual exercise prescription is critical to clinical outcome. Additionally, elderly populations have reduced heat shock protein (HSP) function suggesting that the recovery period between bouts of WBV may be critical.*

Immune function and sarcopenia

Viewing muscle as an organ of the immune system has become a rather novel and intriguing health issue. Tantalizing speculation from an anthropometrical perspective would suggest that as our forebears left the

*Heat shock proteins (HSP) are small proteins, or 'molecular chaperones', considered to be essential for life. They are activated by 'stessors' such as heat and cold, as well as by pathogens (Cubano & Lewis 2001).

Table 3.1 Change in functional performance

Parameter	WBV+		Control n = 11	P^a	P^b
	Initial randomization (n = 13)	Reassessed at 6 weeks (n = 10)			
Chair sit-and-reach (cm)	−20.2 ± 6.2	−21.0 ± 6.9	−23.2 ± 9.4	0.061	0.145
Back scratch (cm)	−23.2 ± 16.0	−23.0 ± 18.3	−15.9 ± 6.9	0.323	0.667
30-second chair stand (number)	6.3 ± 4.0	7.0 ± 4.1	8.2 ± 3.1	0.127	0.303
Tinetti test					
Body balance (score/16)	12.8 ± 3.7	13.4 ± 3.1	13.2 ± 2.6	0.784	0.566
Gait (score/12)	9.6 ± 2.7	9.9 ± 2.8	9.9 ± 2.1	0.891	0.822
Total (score/28)	22.4 ± 5.9	23.3 ± 5.6	23.1 ± 4.3	0.966	0.665
Timed get-up-and-go test (seconds)	17.9 ± 9.3	15.3 ± 5.5	14.8 ± 6.3	0.399	0.743
Grip strength (KPa)	41.6 ± 19.5	43.3 ± 18.9	3.3 ± 24.6	0.765	0.545

Leg extension 40 cm/s					
Work (J)	66.9 ± 74.6	55.8 ± 44.6	88.5 ± 79.4	0.361	0.387
Maximal force (N)	270.0 ± 203.8	251.3 ± 141.4	375.2 ± 253.8	0.277	0.282
Maximal power (W)	108.0 ± 81.5	100.5 ± 56.5	150.1 ± 101.5	0.277	0.282
Maximal explosivity (N/s)	2693.1 ± 1698.3	2755.0 ± 1600.1	4070.0 ± 2483.0	0.134	0.173
Leg extension 60 cm/s					
Work	47.1 ± 57.1	36.9 ± 32.9	68.7 ± 78.6	0.459	0.468
Maximal force (N)	204.3 ± 197.0	178.3 ± 148.1	312.1 ± 281.3	0.283	0.290
Maximal power (W)	123.4 ± 117.4	108.0 ± 87.7	187.3 ± 168.7	0.339	0.359
Maximal explosivity (N/s)	3885.0 ± 3291.6	3553.5 ± 2700.0	4872.3 ± 3371.6	0.424	0.426

Mann-Whitney U test (exact two-tailed significance). Control versus WBV+; [a]initial randomization; [b]reassessed at 6 weeks. Values represent means ± SD. Note the large standard deviations.

Reprinted from Bautmans I, Van Hees E, Lemper J-C et al (2005) The feasibility of whole body vibration in institutionalised elderly persons and its influence on muscle performance, balance and mobility: a randomised controlled trial. *BMC Geriatrics* 5:17 with permission from Tony Mets.

savannahs of Africa they would have required lean muscle mass for practically every aspect of life including hunting, ambulation and even thermoregulation. Additionally, lean muscle mass represented an important sink of protein which the immune system could draw upon when it encountered new pathogens in the regions where they were treading for the very first time. In contrast, modern men and women ambulate far less than previous generations, use air conditioning and central heating for thermoregulation and usually do not go hunting with a spear. Therefore, modern muscle is underutilized and could represent a danger of leaving our other organs to 'fend for themselves'. It is plausible that WBV could represent unique myogenic stimuli which could enhance immune function through the hypertrophy of muscle tissue, activation of HSP, enhanced modulation of cytokines, improved phagocytosis and muscle-induced changes to lymphatic drainage.

WBV training was found to be as efficient as a fitness programme for increasing isometric and explosive knee extension strength and muscle mass of the upper-leg in community-dwelling older men (Bogaerts et al 2007). This is significant as even a 10% loss in lean body mass (LBM) corresponds with impaired immune function (Demling & DeSanti 1997) and a loss of approximately 30% of the body proteins can result in death (Rasmussen & Phillips 2003). During severe trauma, such as burns, the need for essential amino acids drives the catabolic loss of protein from skeletal muscle, which can be as high as 1% per day of illness (Griffiths et al 1999). Accelerated muscle proteolysis is the primary cause of this loss of LBM, which is characteristic of many diseases (Mitch & Goldberg 1996). Some peptides generated by the breakdown of cell proteins are transported to the cell surface where they are presented to cytotoxic lymphocytes, which in turn destroy cells presenting as foreign (e.g. viral) peptides (Mitch & Goldberg 1996). Consequently, successful ageing has been associated with the preservation of muscle mass (Mariani et al 1999) as this would allow these individuals to draw on their store of protein for any infectious–inflammatory–immune responses.

Increased cytokine activity has been associated with ageing and muscle weakness (Ferrucci et al 2002). This age-associated progressive dysregulation of immune response (Apovian 2000) is seen in older women with high interlukin (6) serum levels who have a higher risk of developing physical disability and experience steeper declines in walking ability than those with lower levels (Ferrucci et al 2002). However, the statistical interaction of IL-6 concentration with disability was shown to be non-linear and the progression of disability with IL-6 concentration over time was not investigated (Ferrucci et al 2002). Therefore, it is difficult to conclude whether elevated levels of IL-6 are the cause or the effect of skeletal muscle weakness (Ferrucci et al 2002; Bruunsgaard et al 2003). Furthermore, other authors suggest the IL-6 inhibits TNF-alpha production and insulin resistance (Bruunsgaard et al 2003). Nevertheless, a cycle of inactivity with a chronically impaired inflammatory–immune response is plausible. Therefore, exercise apparatus which stimulates muscle kinetic strength and hence power should inherently enhance cytokine regulation through the anabolic input of enhanced functional capacity.

Blottner et al (2006) used 55 days of bed rest and WBV to demonstrate the preservation of muscle tissue in the soleus muscle. The disrupted pattern of myofibres, with a transformation by up to 140% from type I to type II phenotype (slow to fast twitch), did not occur in the vibration group (Fig. 3.1). Moreover, these researchers were able to demonstrate increased nitrous oxide synthase (NOS) in the soleus muscle of the WBV group (Figs. 3.2 and 3.3). They stated that this was significant as NOS1 is associated with the sarcolemmal dystrophin–glycoprotein complex via

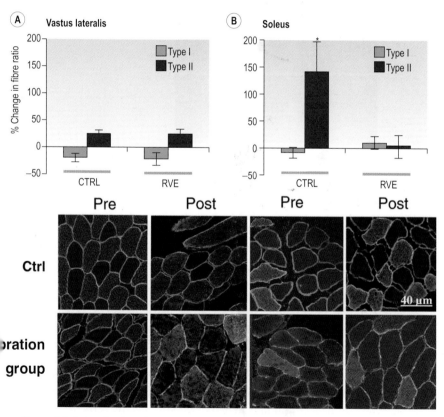

Figure 3.1 Determination of myofibre ratio (type I vs II) in (A) vastus lateralis and (B) Soleus biopsies of the control versus vibration group.

Reprinted from Blottner D, Salanova M, Puttmann B et al (2006) Human skeletal muscle structure and function preserved by vibration muscle exercise following 55 days of bed rest. *European Journal of Applied Physiology* 97:261–271, with permission from Springer.

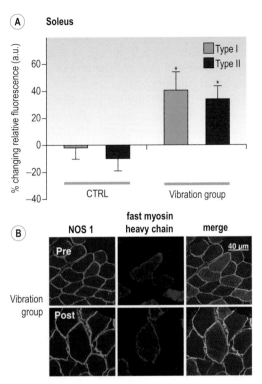

Figure 3.2 (A and B) Expression of muscle fibre activity marker nitrous oxide synthase (NOS1) in subject-matched soleus SOL muscle biopsies.

Reprinted from Blottner D, Salanova M, Puttmann B et al (2006) Human skeletal muscle structure and function preserved by vibration muscle exercise following 55 days of bed rest. *European Journal of Applied Physiology* 97:261–271, with permission from Springer.

syntropin, which is linked to the subsarcolemmal actin network (Bredt 1999).

WBV represents a unique stimulus as its kinetic energy acts directly on the muscle architecture. Similar stimuli such as plyometrics would normally result in broadening and streaming of the Z bands, suggesting muscle damage during eccentric exercise which gives rise to the familiar feeling of delayed-onset muscle soreness (DOMS) with its concomitant release of proinflammatory neurogenic cytokines. This can lead to immobility even in healthy young adults and can be a significant disincentive to exercise. Conversely, unlike eccentric exercise such as plyometrics and progressive resistance training, when applied correctly, WBV represents a milder and more dose-specific form of exercise for the promotion of pro-anabolic hormones for muscle growth which may subsequently aid in the modulation of pro- and anti-inflammatory cytokines.

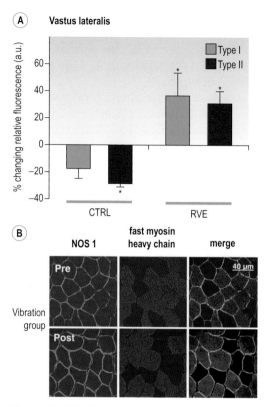

Figure 3.3 (A & B) Expression of muscle fibre activity marker nitrous oxide synthase (NOS1) in subject-matched vastus lateralis muscle biopsies.

Reprinted from Blottner D, Salanova M, Puttmann B et al (2006) Human skeletal muscle structure and function preserved by vibration muscle exercise following 55 days of bed rest. *European Journal of Applied Physiology* 97:261–271 with permission from Springer.

Besides cytokines, HSP have also been implicated in enhanced immune function with regular exercise. Unfortunately, numerous attempts to link exercise to meaningful alterations in immune function have been largely unconvincing (Moseley 2000). It has been argued that it is the local as opposed to the global immune system activation by HSPs which is at the core of immune effects of exercise (Moseley 2000). HSPs are involved in protein folding and sorting, in the assembly of protein complexes and in the binding of denatured proteins, and are primarily induced in response to stress (Puntschart et al 1996). Exercise may provide a hormonal stimulus to regulate HSP proteolysis. Recently, rodent investigations have demonstrated that insulin-like growth factor 1 (IGF-1) inhibits both lysosomal and ubiquitin-proteasome-dependent stress protein breakdown in skeletal muscle (Fang et al 2002), thus suggesting a hormonal regulating mechanism. Significantly, increased IGF-1 concentrations have been demonstrated near the Z bands in the elderly after a resistance training regimen (Urso et al 2001). In particular, eccentric exercises have been associated with damage to these Z bands (Fielding et al 1996). Presumably there is a role for HSP during the recovery from such damage.

In rodents, overloading of atrophied muscles, after a period of immobility, stimulates early increases in IGF-1 in slow twitch oxidative red fibres more than in fast twitch glycolytic white fibres. Release of IGF-1 was considered to be part of the myogenic reactive compensatory process of muscle hypertrophy (Adams et al 1999). IGF-1 induces muscle regulatory factor (MRF), which is facilitated by the inactivation of glycogen synthase kinase (GSK-3beta). This has the potential not only to aid in hypertrophy but also to stimulate myoblastic regrowth (van der Velden et al 2006). In contrast, HSP25 released after muscle overload was greater in the fast twitch plantaris than in the slow twitch soleus, and occurred immediately on overloading and was shown to be greatest between 3 and 7 days post stimuli. Similarly, turmour necrosis factor alpha (TNF-alpha) was increased in the fast twitch plantaris muscle but not in the slow twitch soleus 0.5–2 days after overloading. This last finding was associated with HSP25 in C2C12 myotubes, suggesting greater mechanical stress inflammatory responses in the fast twitch muscles (Huey et al 2007). Therefore, the direct correlation between IGF-1 production in muscle and the regulation of protein synthesis after HSP-induced proteolysis as a result of exercise-induced trauma is tenuous at best. Nevertheless, taken together these investigations demonstrate marked immune reactions within deconditioned muscle after exercise.

Consensus indicates that 'moderate exercise' may enhance immune function and may reduce the incidence of infection while long-term exhaustive exercise results in immunosuppression and an increased susceptibility to infections (Armstrong & VanHeest 2002, Dressendorfer et al 2002, Gleeson 2000, Pedersen et al 1998, Woods et al 1999). This is consistent with Ji (2002), suggesting that the major benefit of non-exhaustive exercise is to induce a mild oxidative stress that stimulates the expression of antioxidant enzymes, as well as the induction of IGF-1 (Fang et al 2002) seen in resistance training (Fiatarone Singh et al 1999, Urso et al 2001). Additionally, resistance training accompanied by nutritional supplementation has been shown to result in significant muscle hypertrophy (Fiatarone et al 1994). Biomechanical principles dictate that, for the same force, the strain in a skeletal muscle is reduced proportional to the skeletal muscle's cross-sectional area (Hunter et al 1998). Therefore, if contractile skeletal muscle mass is maintained or enhanced, then it is plausible that a greater spectrum of 'moderate exercise' can be entertained.

Correctly dosed and progressed WBV probably represents moderate exercise in the vulnerable populations such as the frail elderly, those having undergone prolonged bed rest and people suffering from obesity, diabetes and/or cardiovascular disease. Inflammation and ischaemic reperfusion activates both pro- and anti-apoptotic events in cultured endothelial cells (Yang et al 2006). Ninety minutes of cycling at 2400 m altitude with a 30-Hz, 4-mm amplitude vibration significantly increased vascular endothelial growth factor (VEGF) (Suhr et al 2007). Yang et al (2006) stated that cholesterol-rich, plasma membrane rafts serve an organizational and integrational role in signal transduction which can be activated by oxidative stress. Moreover, HSP27 and HSP70 have been implicated in these inflammatory reactive oxygen species (ROS)-related processes. Rittweger et al (2001) examined oxidative stress, by using 26-Hz, 6-mm WBV to demonstrate increased oxygen consumption of 4.5 mL/min/kg. By using oxygen at 20.9 J/mL = 1.6 W (kg body mass) and walking speed at 0.4 m/s it can be calculated that this requires 2.3 mL/min/kg; therefore 3 min of standing, squatting and holding weights during WBV is metabolically comparable to walking.

Although Cubano and Lewis (2001) using in vitro space flight simulation reported that vibration stress per se had not been shown to affect HSP70, their data demonstrated that vibrated cells underwent an oxidative stress whereby glucose consumption was increased and that a decrease of approximately 30% in RNA for HSP70a/b occurred 48 hours after vibration. When prescribing moderate exercise, these findings may have important implications for the period between doses of WBV. In fact, similar to progressive resistance training (PRT), the consensus may be a stimulus every 72 hours for the treatment of conditions such as metabolic syndrome.

Importantly, WBV is dose-sensitive and can be applied for short periods of time and in varying degrees of weight-bearing using apparatuses such as the tilt table, or by simply loading the body in various positions of knee bend, one- or two-legged standing, with/without free weights. The safety of the methodology can be extrapolated from the data of Roelants et al (2004a) in which after 24 weeks of 35–40-Hz, 2.5–5.0-mm WBV, only one person dropped out due to anterior knee pain compared with six in the PRT group. Similarly, Bautmans et al (2005) demonstrated a 96% completion rate with three times per week for 6 weeks of 30–40 Hz of WBV, and Kawanabe et al (2007) reported no serious adverse events in elderly people during 12–20 Hz, 4 min, once per week over 2 months.

Interestingly, some of the same elements discussed in the previous chapter regarding tensegrity and WBV are also considered to be involved in protection against apoptosis. Oxidants have been shown to impair formation of focal adhesion by stimulating the activity of calpain, leading to degradation of talin and alpha-actinin. Moreover, cell migration requires the involvement of membrane protrusion and the development of new adhesions using actin polymerization and integrin engagement through

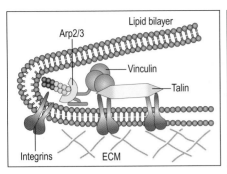 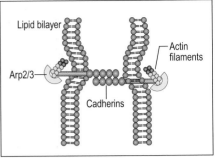

Figure 3.4 Physical coupling of adhesion molecules to the actin polymerization machinery. (Left) The Arp2/3 complex is directly recruited to sites of integrin engagement through an interaction with the linker region of vinculin, an integrin-associated protein. (Right) The Arp2/3 complex is recruited to sites of cell–cell adhesion through an interaction with E-cadherin. Recruitment of the Arp2/3 complex to E-cadherin is thought to localize actin polymerization to sites of cadherin engagement.

Reprinted from DeMali KA, Burridge K (2003) Coupling membrane protrusion and cell adhesion. *Journal of Cell Science* 116(12):2389–2397, with permission from marketing@biologists.com.

transient binding of actin-related protein (Arp2/3) to vinculin (DeMali et al 2002). Together this is significant, as coupling of the membrane protrusions with cell adhesion through cell migration, using cadherin-mediated junction formation, are important elements of phagocytosis seen in the immune system when tissue needs repair (see Fig. 3.4; DeMali & Burridge 2003). Presumably, WBV has the capacity to directly stimulate these cytoskeletal elements as well as stimulate anti-oxidants such as HSP.

Bone

Osteoporosis affects over 25 million Americans alone. It is more prevalent in Caucasian cultures and contributes to morbidity in the increasingly ageing population (Kuruvilla et al 2008). Rittweger (2008) argued strongly for a muscle–bone hypothesis with an intriguing motor control element, restricting maximal load and hence bone density, on articular joint size. Evidence for muscle bone interaction during WBV comes from Verscheuren et al (2004), who found that 6 months of WBV training increased muscle strength and hip bone mineral density (BMD) in postmenopausal women. Skerry (2008) argued that a single saturating load of only 72 s will load the bone sufficiently to produce a maximal osteogenic loading response. This was based on the work by Rubin and Lanyon (1984), in which they showed that 8 s of loading, four times in a 24 hour period, was sufficient to produce maximum bone loading response in the wings of chickens. Moreover, it was suggested that, if a single loading cycle is repeated in two, three or four separate bouts, then this effect is not only sustained but enables long-term potentiation through glutamate signaling (Fig. 3.5; Skerry 2008). Further research by Rubin et al (2001) using a 28-day hind-limb suspension protocol in mice confirmed that disuse alone resulted in a 92% reduction in bone formation rates, which reduced to 61% if this was interrupted by 10 min weight-bearing, but moreover this reduction was completely normalized with 10 min of 90-Hz, 0.25-g vibration therapy. This has important implications for people undergoing long periods of bed rest.

When reconsidering the tensegrity model, the repeated loading of WBV could be representing enhanced pre-tension on trabecular structure through the effect of vibration on bone rheology. Jordan (2005) considered bone perfusion to correlate with bone density. However, Cardinale

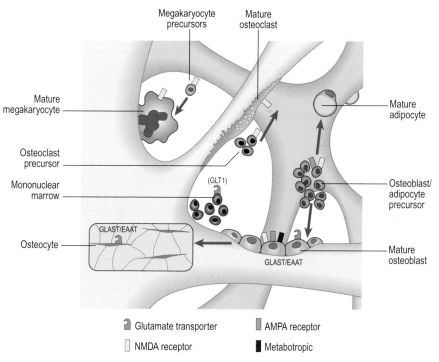

Figure 3.5 Sites of expression of components of the glutamatergic signalling mechanism within bone. Osteoblasts express pre- and postsynaptic components and glutamate, whereas osteoclasts, osteocytes and megakaryocytes express a more restricted subset of post synaptic receptor components (Skerry 2008).
NMDA = N-methyl-D-aspartate
AMPA = α-amino-3-hydroxyl-5-methyl-4-isoxazole-propionate

Reprinted from *Trends in Pharmacological Sciences* 22/4, Skerry and Genever (2001), with permission from Elsevier.

et al (2007) found little difference in medial gastrocnemius and vastus lateralis muscle perfusion after 110 s of static squatting using 30-, 40- and 50-Hz WBV in young men. Conversely, Stewart et al (2004) used peri-menopausal women, tilted at 35°, to demonstrate 20–35% enhancements in blood flow in the calf (30%), pelvis (26%) and thoracic regions (20%) with 45-Hz, $2g$, 2-m^2 (vertical displacements 25 μm) WBV. Hypoxia together with vibration-induced shear stress was demonstrated to induce angiogenesis during 90 min high intensity cycling at altitude with 30-Hz (4-mm) WBV (Suhr et al 2007). Since the tensegrity model requires fluid to counterbalance the tensile elements it is worthy of speculation that increased perfusion would positively influence bone mass.

Since WBV can be shown to improve functional capacity in the SF-36 (Bruyere et al 2005), then this enhanced activity alone should improve BMD. More importantly, for the bed-ridden person any training regimen which prevents and/or attenuates the loss of muscle mass and bone density should improve quality of life. Belavý et al (2008) used WBV of 19–26 Hz, with amplitude 3.5–4 mm, 1.2–1.8g, to reduce lumbar spine multifidus deconditioning with bed rest. WBV of 18 Hz, using explosive squats-in-supine, prevented bed rest atrophy and improved maximal amplitude on electromyogram by 30% from day 10 onwards. However, this was task-specific at the peripheral motor unit site and hence did not prevent task-non-specific loss of function (Mulder et al 2007).

Clinical effects of WBV on bone density

Gusi et al (2006) demonstrated in their WBV group BMD femoral neck increases of 4.3% more than in their walking group. However, BMD of the lumbar spine remained unaltered in both groups. Judex et al (2007) used ovariectomized rats to demonstrate greater trabecular volume (22 and 25%) and thicker trabecular structure (11 and 12%) in the epiphysis of the distal femur at 90-Hz WBV compared with 45-Hz, despite strain rates and magnitudes being significantly lower at 90 Hz than at 45 Hz (Fig. 3.6). Extrapolation to humans would need to consider the effect of muscle resistance on the amplitude of oscillations. As muscles contract, they would generate greater stiffness, thereby damping the amplitude of oscillation. Iwamato et al (2005) demonstrated no difference in BMD but their training stimuli was only 20 Hz, once per week, lasting 4 min.

Additional investigations carried out on animals which need mention-ing are those by Flieger et al (1998), who conducted trials over 12 weeks with ovariectomized rats. The rats were they placed under vibration at a

Fluorescence microscopy   Polarization microscopy

Sham

OVX
Vib 45Hz

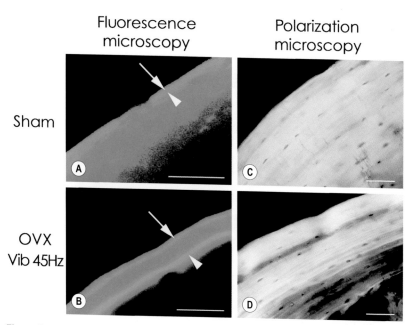

Figure 3.6 Microphotos of undecalcified cortical bone cross-sections prepared from mid-diaphyseal tibiae of 1-year-old female rats submitted to ovariectomy (OVX) and vertical vibration [WBV 45 Hz (3.0*g*), 30 min/day for 90 days]. The sections were studied by fluorescence microscopy (A and B, original magnification ×250) and by polarization microscopy (C and D, original magnification ×250). Calcein was injected at day 63 (arrowhead) and tetracycline at day 84 (arrow). The polarization microscopy showed lamellar bone, formed and located circumferentially during the labelling period. Horizontal bars = 50 μm.
Reprinted from *Bone* 32/1, Oxlund et al (2003), with permission from Elsevier.

frequency of 50 Hz, amplitude 2*g* for 30 min every day. These authors found that the experimental group had significantly less bone loss than the sham group and the control group. Oxlund et al (2003) also studied the effect of low-intensity and high-frequency vibration on bone mass, bone strength and skeletal muscle mass in the adult ovariectomized rat model, by comparing different vibration frequencies, 17 Hz (0.5*g*), 30 Hz (1.5*g*) and 45 Hz (3.0*g*), with a control group and a sham group. Vibrations, with amplitude of 1.0 mm, were given for 30 min every day for a total of 90 days (Fig. 3.6). The result was that vibration at 45 Hz increased periosteal bone formation rate, inhibited the endocortical bone resorption and inhibited the decline in maximum bending stress and compressive stress induced by the ovariectomization. Vibration did not influence the skeletal muscle mass. One can note that this is in agreement with Rubin's findings, which supports the idea of a possible direct beneficial effect of this kind of treatment on the preservation of bone (Figs 3.7 and 3.8).

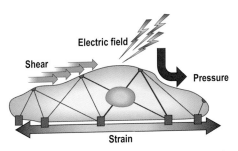

Figure 3.7 Mechanical force in the cellular environment.
Reprinted from *Gene* 367, Rubin et al (2006), with permission from Elsevier.

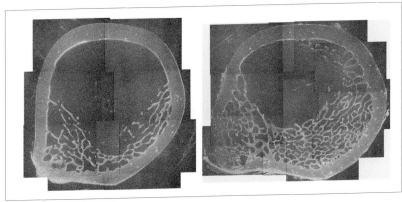

Figure 3.8 Mechanical input from 20 min per day of 30 Hz of 0.3g mechanical vibration for 1 year improves trabecular structure.
Reprinted from *Gene* 367, Rubin et al (2006), with permission from Elsevier.

Clinical effects of WBV on obesity and metabolic syndrome

Obesity significantly exacerbates the deleterious effect of diabetes, dyslipidemia and hypertension. Regular exercise involving energy expenditure has been advocated by various health authorities to tackle obesity. Similarly, regular exercise can improve muscle mass, which is an important 'sink' for the action of insulin. Importantly, the convenience and comfort of exercise are variables which influence training programme compliance. WBV is a time-efficient and convenient method of training.

Rittweger et al (2001, 2002) calculated the energy consumptions of various exercises with WBV and compared these with walking. Vibration elicits a metabolic muscular response and therefore is not a passive form of exercise. During 3 min of WBV training oxygen consumption increased by 4.5 mL/min/kg. Using oxygen at 20.9 J/mL = 1.6 W (kg body mass) it can be calculated that walking speed at 0.4 m/s requires 2.3 mL/min/kg, which means that WBV is metabolically comparable to walking in an elderly frail population. Using 18–34-Hz, 5-mm amplitude, with the addition of 40% lean body mass attached to waist and later shoulders, achieved a linear and significant increase in oxygen consumption from 18 to 34 Hz; at 26 Hz the oxygen consumption increased more than proportionally with amplitudes increasing from 2.5 to 7.5 mm (Rittweger et al 2002). Roelants et al (2004b) used 24 weeks of WBV to achieve a fat-free mass (FFM) increase of 2.2%. Significant increases in strength in WBV of 24.4 ± 5.1% and in a training group of 16.5 ± 1.7% were also shown.

Animal studies (Rubin et al 2007) using 5 days per week, 15 min of 0.2g, 90-Hz WBV found inhibition of adipogenesis by 27%, reduced nonesterified free fatty acid and triglycerides by 43 and 39%. Over 9 weeks fat production was suppressed by 22% in chemically (C3H.B6-6T) accelerated age-related mice. Mesenchymal stem cell differentiation into adipocytes reduced by 19%. However, it is difficult to make a direct clinical comparison as the training dose used was double that used in humans. Until further investigations are made, it would seem that, in the absence of contraindications, the WBV training therapy would be an appropriate approach when one considers the morbidity and socio economic costs associated with metabolic syndrome.

Conclusion

Although many questions remain, this chapter highlights some of the potential sites of action of WBV. These include the direct training affect of WBV in maintaining and improving muscle mass which may act as a metabolic & immune organ important for survival. However, the direct effects of WBV on immune function remain highly speculative. Nevertheless, enhanced quality of daily functional activities due to increased strength would intuitively improve the body as a whole. Furthermore, the effects of WBV on blood flow & bone mineral density suggest an important role in the prevention & treatment of osteoporosis. Taken together these studies attempt to describe the construct validity for future research based on a receptor and molecular level of the potential effects of WBV in the treatment and prevention of morbidity issues associated with aging. Clinically, practitioners now have a new horizon to explore whereby improvements in their clinical outcomes are the ultimate goal when working with 'at risk' sedentary and aging populations. In this manner practice based evidence and evidence based practice can evolve together to determine the usefulness of WBV.

References

Adams GR, Haddad F, Baldwin KM (1999) Time course of changes in markers of myogenesis in overloaded rat skeletal muscles. *Journal of Applied Physiology* 87(5):1705–1712.

Apovian CM (2000) Nutrition and aging. *Current Opinion in Endocrinology, Diabetes and Obesity* 7(5):231–235.

Armstrong LE, VanHeest JL (2002) The unknown mechanism of the overtraining syndrome clues from depression and psychoneuroimmunology. *Sports Medicine* 32:185–209.

Bautmans I, Van Hees E, Lemper J-C et al (2005) The feasibility of whole body vibration in institutionalised elderly persons and its influence on muscle performance, balance and mobility: a randomised controlled trial. *BMC Geriatrics* 5:17.

Belavý DL, Hides JA, Wilson SJ et al (2008) Resistive simulated weight bearing exercise with whole body vibration reduces lumbar spine deconditioning in bed-rest. *Spine* 33(5):121–131.

Blottner D, Salanova M, Puttmann B et al (2006) Human skeletal muscle structure and function preserved by vibration muscle exercise following 55 days of bed rest. *European Journal of Applied Physiology* 97:261–271.

Bogaerts A, Delecluse C, Claessens AL et al (2007) Impact of whole-body vibration training versus fitness training on muscle strength and muscle mass in older men. A 1-year randomized controlled trial. *Journal of Gerontology and Medical Sciences* 62(6):630–635.

Bredt D (1999) Endogenous nitric oxide synthesis: biological functions and pathophysiology. *Free Radical Research* 31:577–596.

Bruunsgaard H, Ladelund S, Pedersen AN et al (2003) Predicting death from tumour necrosis factor alpha and interleukin 6 in 80-year-old people. *Clinical and Experimental Immunology* 132:24–31.

Bruyere O, Wuidart M-A, Di Palma E et al (n.d.) Controlled whole body vibrations to decrease fall risk and improve health related quality of life in elderly patients. Conference presentation, World Health Organization.

Bruyere O, Wuidart M-A, Di Palma E et al (2005) Controlled whole body vibration to decrease fall risk and improve health-related quality of life of nursing home residents. *Archives of Physical Medicine and Rehabilitation* 86:303–307.

Cardinale M, Ferrari M, Quaresima V (2007) Gastrocnemius medialis and vastus lateralis oxygenation during whole body vibration exercise. *Medicine and Science in Sports and Exercise* 39(4):694–700.

Cheung WH, Mok HW, Qin L et al (2007) High-frequency whole-body vibration improves balancing ability in elderly women. *Archives of Physical Medicine and Rehabilitation* 88(7):852–857.

Cubano LA, Lewis ML (2001) Effects of vibrational stress and spaceflight on regulation of heat shock proteins hsp70 and hsp27 in human lymphocytes (Jurkat). *Journal of Leukocyte Biology* 69:755–761.

DeMali KA, Burridge K (2003) Coupling membrane protrusion and cell adhesion. *Journal of Cell Science* 116(12):2389–2397.

DeMali KA, Barlow C A, Burridge K (2002) Recruitment of the Arp2/3 complex to vinculin: coupling membrane protrusion to matrix adhesion. *Journal of Cell Biology* 159(5):881–891.

Demling RH, DeSanti L (1997) Oxandrolone, an anabolic steroid significantly increases the rate of weight gain in the recovery phase after major burns. *Journal of Trauma: Injury, Infection, and Critical Care* 43:47–51.

Dressendorfer RH, Petersen SR, Moss Lovshin SE et al (2002) Performance enhancement with maintenance of resting immune status after intensified cycle training. *Clinical Journal of Sport Medicine* 12:301–307.

Fang CH, Li BG, Wray CJ et al (2002) Insulin-like growth factor-I inhibits lysosomal and proteasome-dependent proteolysis in skeletal muscle after burn injury. *Journal of Burn Care and Rehabilitation* 23:318–325.

Ferrucci L, Penninx BW, Volpato S et al (2002) Change in muscle strength explains accelerated decline of physical function in older women with high interleukin 6 serum levels. *Journal of the American Geriatrics Society* 50:1947–1954.

Fiatarone MA, O'Neill EF, Ryan ND et al (1994) Exercise training and nutritional supplementation for physical frailty in very elderly people. *New England Journal of Medicine* 330:1769–1775.

Fiatarone Singh MA, Ding W, Manfredi TJ et al (1999) Insulin-like growth factor I in skeletal muscle after weight-lifting exercise in frail elders. *American Journal of Physiology—Endocrinology and Metabolism* 277:E135–E143.

Fielding RA, Manfredi T, Parzick A et al (1996) Eccentric exercise induced muscle injury in humans. *Medicne and Science in Sports and Exercise* 28:188.

Flieger J, Karachalios Th, Khaidi P et al (1998) Mechanical Stimulation in the form of vibration prevents postmenopausal bone loss in Ovariectomized Rats. *Calcif Tissue Int* 63:510–514.

Gleeson M (2000) Overview: exercise immunology. *Immunology and Cell Biology* 78:483–484.

Griffiths RD, Hinds CJ, Little RA (1999) Manipulating the metabolic response to injury. *British Medical Bulletin* 55:181–195.

Gusi N, Raimundo A, Leal A (2006) Low frequency vibratory exercise reduces the risk of bone fracture more than walking: a randomized controlled trial. *BMC Musculoskeletal Disorders* 7(92):1–8.

Huey KA, McCall GE, Zhong H et al (2007) Modulation of HSP25 and TNF-alpha during the early stages of functional overload of a rat slow and fast muscle. *Journal of Applied Physiology* 102:2307–2314.

Hunter SM, White M, Thompson M (1998) Techniques to evaluate elderly human muscle function: a physiological basis. *Journals of Gerontology Series A Biological Sciences and Medical Sciences* 53A:204–216.

Ingber DE (2006) Cellular mechanotransduction: putting all the pieces together again. *FASEB Journal* 20:811–827.

Iwamato J, Takeda T, Sato Y et al (2005) Effect of whole-body vibration exercise on lumbar bone mineral density, bone turnover, and chronic back pain in post-menopausal osteoporotic women treated with alendronate. *Aging Clinical and Experimental Research* 17(2):157–163.

Ji LL (2002) Exercise-induced modulation of antioxidant defense. *Annals of the New York Academy of Sciences* 959:82–92.

Jordan J (2005) Good vibrations and strong bones. *American Journal of Physiology: Integrated Comparative Physiology* 288:555–556.

Judex S, Lei X, Han C et al (2007) Low-magnitude mechanical signals that stimulate bone formation in the ovariectomized rat are dependent on the applied frequency but not on the strain magnitude. *Journal of Biomechanics* 40(6):1333–1339.

Kawanabe K, Kawashima A, Sashimoto I et al (2007) Effect of whole-body vibration exercise and muscle strengthening on walking ability in the elderly. *Keio Journal of Medicine* 56(1):28–33.

Kuruvilla SJ, Fox SD, Cullen DM et al (2008) Site specific bone adaptation response to mechanical loading. *Journal of Musculoskeletal and Neuronal Interactions* 8(1):71–78.

Mariani E, Ravaglia G, Forti P et al (1999) Vitamin D, thyroid hormones and muscle mass influence natural killer NK innate immunity in healthy nonagenarians and centenarians. *Clinical and Experimental Immunology* 116:19–27.

Mitch WE, Goldberg AL (1996) Mechanisms of disease mechanisms of muscle wasting the role of the ubiquitin-proteasome pathway. *New England Journal of Medicine* 335:1897–1905.

Morley JE, Baumgartner RN, Roubenoff R et al (2001) Sarcopenia. *Journal of Laboratory and Clinical Medicine* 137:231–243.

Moseley P (2000) Exercise stress and the immune conversation. *Exercise and Sport Sciences Reviews* 28:128–132.

Mulder ER, Gerrits KHL, Kleine BU et al (2007) High intensity surface EMG study on the time course of central nervous and peripheral neuromuscular changes during 8 weeks of bed rest with or without resistive vibration exercise. *Journal of Electromyography and Kinesiology* 19(2):208–218.

Oxlund BS, Ørtoft G, Andreassena TT et al (2003) Low-intensity, high-frequency vibration appears to prevent the decrease in strength of the femur and tibia associated with ovariectomy of adult rats. *Bone* 32:69–77.

Pedersen BK, Rohde T, Ostrowski K (1998) Recovery of the immune system after exercise. *Acta Physiologica Scandinavica* 162:325–332.

Puntschart A, Vogt M, Widmer HR et al (1996) Hsp70 expression in human skeletal muscle after exercise. *Acta Physiologica Scandinavica* 157:411–417.

Rasmussen BB, Phillips SM (2003) Contractile and nutritional regulation of human muscle growth. *Exercise and Sport Sciences Reviews* 31:127–131.

Rittweger J (2008) Ten years muscle-bone hypothesis: what have we learned so far almost a festschrift. *Journal of Musculoskeletal and Neuronal Interactions* 8(2):174–178.

Rittweger J, Schiessl H, Felsenberg D (2001) Oxygen uptake during whole-body vibration exercise: comparison with squatting as a slow voluntary movement. *European Journal of Applied Physiology* 86:169–173.

Rittweger J, Ehrig J, Just K et al (2002) Oxygen uptake during whole-body vibration exercise: influence of vibration frequency, amplitude, and external load. *International Journal of Sports Medicine* 23:428–432.

Roelants M, Delecluse C, Verschueren SM (2004a) Whole-body-vibration training increases knee-extension strength and speed of movement in older women. *Journal of the American Geriatric Society* 52:901–908.

Roelants M, Delecluse C, Goris M et al (2004b) Effects of 24 weeks of whole body vibration training on body composition and muscle strength in untrained females. *International Journal of Sports Medicine* 25(1):1–5.

Rosenberg IH, Roubenoff R (1995) Stalking sarcopenia. *Annals of Internal Medicine* 23:727–728.

Rubin CT, Lanyon LE (1984) Regulation of bone formation by applied dynamic loads. *Journal of Bone and Joint Surgery, American* 66A:397–402.

Rubin C, Xu G, Judex S (2001) The anabolic activity of bone tissue suppressed by disuse is normalized by brief exposure to extremely low-magnitude mechanical stimuli. *FASEB Journal* 15:225–229.

Rubin CT, Capilla E, Luu YK et al (2007) Adipogenesis is inhibited by brief daily exposure to high frequency extremely low-magnitude mechanical signals. *Proceedings of the National Academy of Sciences of the United States of American* 104(45):17879–17884.

Rubin J, Rubin C, Jacobs CR (2006) Molecular pathways mediating mechanical signaling in bone. *Gene* 367:1–16.

Skerry TM (2008) The role of glutamate in the regulation of bone mass and architecture. *Journal of Musculoskeletal and Neuronal Interactions* 8(2):166–173.

Skerry JM, Genever P (2001) Glutamate signalling in non-neuronal tissues. *Trends Pharmacol Sci* 22:174–181.

Stewart JM, Karman C, Montgomery LD et al (2004) Plantar vibration improves leg fluid flow in perimenopausal women. *American Journal of Physiology: Regulatory, Integrative and Comparative Physiology* 288:623–629.

Suhr F, Brixius K, de Marées M, et al (2007) Effects of short-term vibration and hypoxia during high-intensity cycling exercise on circulating levels of angiogenic regulators in humans. *Journals of Applied Physiology* 103:474–483.

Sultan C, Stamenovic D, Ingber DE (2004) A computational tensegrity model predicts dynamic rheological behaviours in living cells. *Annals of Biomedical Engineering* 32(4):520–530.

Urso ML, Manfredi TMF, Fiatarone MA (2001) Skeletal muscle IGF-I receptor localization and quantitation following resistance training in the frail elderly. *Medicine and Science in Sports and Exercise* 33:187.

van der Velden JLJ, Langren RCJ, Kelders MCJM et al (2006) Myogenic differentiation during regrowth of atrophied skeletal muscle is associated with inactivation of GSK-3beta. *American Journal of Physiology: Cell Physiology* 292:1636–1644.

Verscheuren SMP, Roelants M, Delecluse C et al (2004) Effect of 6 month whole body vibration training on hip density, muscle strength and postural control in postmenopausal women a randomized controlled pilot study. *Journal of Bone and Mineral Research* 19(3):352–359.

Woods JA, Lowder TW, Keylock KT (1999) Exercise and cellular innate immune function. *Medicine and Science in Sports and Exercise* 31:57–66.

Yang B, Oo TN, Rizzo V (2006) Lipid rafts mediate H202 prosurvival effects in cultured endothelial cells. *FASEB Journal* 20:E688–E697.

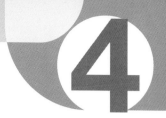

Indications and contraindications in the clinical application of WBV

Immediate and long-term effects and their influence on the selection of dosage

Alfio Albasini and Martin Krause

Indications

Whole body vibration (WBV) has been advocated for:

- Improvement in function
  - get up and go (GUG) test;
  - balance;
  - counter movement jumping;
  - muscle power;
  - muscle length;
  - muscle strength; and
  - motor control.
- Improvement and/or amelioration of specific conditions
  - sarcopenia;
  - osteopenia;
  - stroke;
  - parkinson's disease;
  - diabetes;
  - fibromyalgia;
  - prevention of bed rest-induced muscle atrophy;
  - low back pain; and
  - prevention of injury

Contraindications

WBV may be considered harmful in people with conditions such as:

- pregnancy;
- acute thrombosis;
- serious cardiovascular disease;
- pacemaker;
- recent wounds from an accident or surgery;
- hip and knee implants;
- acute hernia, discopathy, spondylolysis;
- severe diabetes;
- epilepsy;
- recent infections;
- severe migraine;
- tumors;
- recently placed intrauterine devices, metal pins or plates;
- kidney stones;
- organ failure; and
- clinical conditions in which WBV is not indicated.

Clinical research on acute and long-term effects of WBV

Clinical research into the acute and long-term effects of WBV gives us some construct and predictive clinical validity as to the dosage of WBV under various conditions. Despite the scientific evidence on the benefits of vibration training, one must be aware that there are several variables which need to be taken into consideration when interpreting the current and past results reported in the literature. One of the most important factors is the variability in the prescription of dosage as well as the protocols used by different investigators in WBV training, which make direct comparisons difficult and lead to inconsistent results, thereby making conclusions derived from randomized controlled trials (RCTs) complicated. However, this variability gives the clinician an insight into determining the appropriate populations for using WBV through the predicted clinical outcome which then can define the clinical reasoning process.

Vibration protocols can vary in the characteristic of the vibration (vertical vs rotational) as well as the frequency employed. Abercromby et al (2007a) in their study determined the effects of static and dynamic squatting, muscle contraction type using two types of vibration direction, rotational vibration (RV) and vertical vibration (VV) and removing large vibration-induced artefacts from EMG data which is what they also proposed as conclusion of the study. They found that the average responses of the extensors were significantly greater during RV than VV, whereas responses of the tibialis anterior were significantly greater during VV than RV. In their second study, Abercromby et al (2007b) evaluated quantitatively vibration exposure and biodynamic responses during typical WBVT regimens using two different types of vibration, as in the previous study, rotational vibration (RV) and vertical vibration (VV). The key finding of this study was that the risk of adverse health effects would be lower on a short duration exposures to RV (rotational vibration) than VV (vertical vibration) and at half-squats (small knee flexion angle 26-30°) rather than full-squats or upright stance. Furthermore, the parameter of amplitude also varies widely and frequently remains undefined. The duration of the exposure on the platform and the length of time between the cessation of the vibration exposure and the commencement of post-treatment measurements are other important factors which can modify the outcome of the clinical results. Additional variables include the position of the body during WBV, the degree of muscle contraction which can affect the biological response to vibration (Griffin 1997) and the specific movements tested following the vibration treatment.

As the populations using WBV vary markedly, so do the outcome measures. It has been reported that WBV may be an effective intervention for warming up for athletic events as well as for general exercise regimen (Cochrane et al 2007, Jordan et al 2005). Other investigations report significant improvements in disability and vitality measures in institutionalized elderly people (Bautmans et al 2005, Bruyere et al 2005, Kawanabe et al 2007, Roelants et al 2004a,b), while others have reported improvement in measures of strength in animals (Rubin et al 2007), blood flow (Stewart et al 2004) and bone mineral density (BMD) (Verschueren et al 2004) in post- and perimenopausal women. Additionally, neurological conditions such as Parkinson's disease (Haas et al 2006), multiple sclerosis (Schuhfried et al 2005) and stroke (van Nes et al 2004) have also been treated with WBV. Hereby, it can be seen that the populations using WBV vary widely, which makes comparisons difficult. Nevertheless, what can be gleaned from these investigations is that a frequency of <20 Hz is used for muscle relaxation, whereas those between 26 and 44 Hz are used for improving issues related to muscle power and strength. Stimulation to the lower limbs above 50 Hz is thought to cause severe muscle damage (Rittweger et al 2002a). Duration generally does not exceed 10 min, in which the total initial stimulation is in the order of a few minutes with breaks between repetitions. Thus, the duration is progressive and incremental, depending upon the clinical outcomes being achieved.

Acute effects of WBV using the variables of duration, frequency, body positioning and amplitude

Most of the investigations to date have concentrated on the effect of WBV on functional neuromuscular performance in terms of muscle power and strength. In particular counter movement jump (CMJ), vertical jump, running speed and balance have been used as outcome measures. Other measures of the acute effects of WBV were taken using hormonal concentrations and cardiovascular changes. Moreover, the acute effects of WBV vary, depending upon the loading capacity and condition of the individual. Therefore, the dosage prescribed must be safe while still representing an efficacious loading for stimulating anabolic responses to the musculoskeletal system.

Amplitude and frequency

Rittweger et al (2002b) investigated the effect of frequency and demonstrated that vibration at an amplitude of 5 mm was accompanied by a linear increase in oxygen consumption from 18 to 34 Hz and that at 26 Hz the oxygen consumption increased more than proportionally with amplitudes from 2.5 to 7.5 mm.

Bruyere et al (2005) used peak-to-peak amplitudes of 3 and 7 mm with 10 and 26 Hz using a crossover design in institutionalized elderly. A vertically oscillating platform was used to determine the optimal WBV stimulus (frequency × amplitude), 2 and 4 mm at 25, 30, 35, 40 and 45 Hz. Unfortunately these authors did not report specifically on any variation in effect of these changes in parameters, and ideally the amplitude should have been changed without any changes in frequencies to really determine the effect. Nevertheless, it was found that higher WBV amplitude (4 mm) and frequencies (35, 40, 45 Hz) resulted in the greatest increases in electromyogram (EMG) activity (increase in vastus lateralis by 2.9–6.7% in static and 3.7–8.7% under dynamic conditions: Hazell et al 2007).

Body positioning and fatigue

Body positioning and its acute effects is another parameter which can define the prescription of dose. A person standing on a platform requires muscle activation from the lower limbs in order to dampen the vibrations coming up from the vibrating plate (Rubin et al 2003, Wakeling et al 2002). Using intramedullary pins in the greater trochanter and L4 vertebra, researchers were able to demonstrate decreased transmissibility of vibration with varying postures. In relaxed stance transmissibility reduced to 30%, with 20° knee flexion transmissibility reduced to 30%. Additionally, a phase-lag, as high as 70°, occurred between the hips and lumbar spine (Rubin et al 2003). In this study, a unique vibration platform developed for use in a clinical setting was used to impose the WBV. The platform was driven to provide a force of 36Np_p at all loading frequencies, with data collection recorded at 2 Hz, intervals at 15 Hz and finishing at 35 Hz. Rittweger et al (2001) measured an increase in the rate of oxygen consumption during the exposure to vibration. During this research, these investigators not only utilized WBV training but also added dynamic changes in body position in addition to extra loads of up to 40% of the subject's body weight at their waists until exhaustion. Rittweger et al (2001) tested 37 young healthy subjects standing with their feet 15 cm away from the axis of rotation on either side of a platform with a horizontal displacement. Vibration frequency of 26 Hz and a peak acceleration force of $15g$ were used. The authors compared two WBV exercise sessions with bicycle ergometry. Heart rate, blood pressure and oxygen uptake and perceived exertion on Borg's scale increased. Systolic arterial blood pressure and heart rate were found to have increased after WBV but less so than after bicycle ergometry. In contrast, diastolic blood pressure had decreased only after WBV. However, after WBV, jump height was reduced by 9.1%, voluntary force in knee extension reduced by 9.2% and the reduced muscle electromyography (mEMG) during maximal voluntary contraction was attenuated. Taking these results together, one can hypothesize that there are probably two mechanisms of fatigue a neural one and a muscular one. Furthermore, this demonstrates that WBV elicits a metabolic muscular response and therefore is not a passive form of exercise. Oxygen consumption is increased 4.5 mL/min/kg Rittweger et al (2001); this is comparable to walking at 0.4 m/s, which requires 2.3 mL/min/kg.

Muscle function

Torvinen et al (2002a), using a randomized crossover design, tested 16 young adults to investigate a 4-min vibration bout on muscle performance and body balance. A tilting plate, Galileo, was utilized for the intervention where the subjects were asked to stand in different manners. These included a relaxed position, light squatting, on the heels, light jumping and alternating the body weight from one leg to another. The vibration frequency increased in 1-min intervals from 15 Hz by the first minute to 30 Hz for the last minute. The test was performed on 2 days, WBV versus non-WBV, or sham-loading. The peak-to-peak amplitude was 10 mm, with a maximal acceleration of $3.5g$ (where g is the Earth's gravitational field or 9.81 m/s^2). Six performance tests were conducted 10 min before (baseline), and 2 and 60 min after the intervention. Bipolar surface EMG from soleus, gastrocnemius and vastus lateralis muscles were recorded during the 4-min bout of WBV intervention. The vibration loading, based on the Galileo tilting plate, induced a transient increase (especially on the 2-min test) in the isometric extension strength of the lower extremities by 3.2% ($p = 0.020$), a 2.5% ($p = 0.019$) benefit in the jump height and a 15.7% improvement in the body balance ($p = 0.049$). Interestingly, these effects were seen at 2 min, but had disappeared more or less completely after 1 hour. A decrease EMG mean power frequency (mpf) of all muscles during the vibration was seen, indicating that a long-term irritation of the muscle-spindle by vibration leads to muscle fatigue (Eklund 1972).

In another study, Issurin and Tenenbaum (1999) examined 14 elite and 14 amateur athletes who were subjected to vibratory stimulation during bilateral biceps curl exercises using explosive strength exertion. Each subject performed two separate series of three sets of bilateral biceps curls in random order. In the second set of one series, a vibration stimulus was administered through a cable to the handle and therefore to the arm muscle. The stimulus frequency was 44 Hz with an amplitude of 3 mm. Elite and amateur athletes showed an improvement of 10.4 and 7.9%, respectively, in maximal power attributed to vibratory stimulation. In contrast, 65-Hz stimulation directly to the biceps tendon reduced neuromuscular performance (Moran et al 2007). Hence, frequencies of <50 Hz are used.

Hormones and muscle function

Carmelo Bosco, Marco Cardinale and colleagues conducted several investigations over the past several years whereby they reported that WBV interventions would enhance strength and power in well-trained people. Besides the improvements in muscular power, in his PhD thesis, Cardinale (2002) also demonstrated that WBV produces an immediate effect on hormone levels. These results included increased testosterone by 7%, increased growth hormone by 460% and reduced cortisol by 32%. The last finding suggests that WBV is not a stressful experience in physically active individuals, when the 10-min protocol was subdivided into two sets of five subsets, lasting 1 min each with a 6-min rest between sets. However, when a protocol of 7 min of constant WBV was used, vertical jumping ability actually declined and cortisol concentrations actually rose. Therefore, precise dosage in terms of sets and rest periods are important.

Bosco et al (1999a) evaluated the influence of vibration on the mechanical properties of arm flexors, in a group of 12 international-level boxers. The experiment consisted of five repetitions lasting 1 min each with mechanical vibration (30 Hz, 6-mm displacement). The results showed an increase in power output by 12% in unilateral bicep curl. Investigating the lower extremity, Bosco et al (1999b) demonstrated that 10 min (10 times 60 s) of whole body vibration training (WBVT) at 26 Hz with 10-mm peak-to-peak amplitude, on well-trained volleyball players, improved vertical jumping ability. In a follow-up investigation, in young men, they demonstrated increased concentrations of testosterone and growth hormone and also decreases in the blood concentration of the body's stress hormone, cortisol (Bosco et al 2000).

These astonishing results on hormones have been used, and abused, by various companies to promote WBVT and exercises as well as to sell WBV platforms, as 'it boosts hormones, like testosterone and growth hormone, and reduces cortisol and stress whilst enhancing muscle remodelling.' One should not lose sight of the fact that there are also numerous studies which do not show any improvement in strength/power performance and hormone concentrations. Additionally, several limitations of these studies include small numbers ($n = 6$, 12 and 14), with the latter not randomly assigned and therefore without a control group. Bosco et al (1999a,b) also did not indicate in either study the duration between the WBVT and the measurements of their effect, which is essential information for the reproducibility of these results in future trials.

Two investigations, by De Ruiter et al (2003a) and Di Loreto et al (2004), demonstrated no improvement with WBVT. In the work of De Ruiter et al (2003a), subjects exercised on a vibration platform using five sets of 1 min with a frequency of 30 Hz and amplitude of 8 mm, but with 2 min rest between sets. The result showed a reduction in maximal voluntary knee extension force. Of note is the difference in the protocol, in which the 2-min rest period between sets is quite different from other studies. Di Loreto et al (2004) did not notice any change in serum concentrations of growth hormone insulin-like growth factor 1 (IGF-1) and free and total testosterone. In their investigation, WBVT was performed for 10 min at 30 Hz albeit using relatively small amplitude. Since no change in serum levels of IGF-1 could be seen, investigations of intramuscular IGF-1 may be more beneficial in determining a muscular growth-stimulating effect. On a positive note, Di Loreto et al (2004) did find that vibration slightly reduced plasma glucose (30 min: vibration 4.59 ± 0.21, control 4.74 ± 0.22 nM, $p = 0.049$) and increased plasma norepinephrine concentrations (60 min: vibration 1.29 ± 0.18, control 1.01 ± 0.07 nM, $p = 0.038$).

Swelling and erythema

Swelling and erythema of the foot after WBV, particularly in the first session and especially in women, was observed by Rittweger et al (2000). Also itching was reported frequently, but these changes resolved rapidly if the subjects walked around. The question that arises is whether the swelling and erythema are caused by vasodilation of supplying arteries via an increase in perfusion pressure or whether it is a direct mechanical effect. Since the oedema and erythema were observed on the plantar surfaces of the feet, i.e. the body part closest to the vibrating platform, Rittweger et al (2000) concluded that the explanation was a direct mechanical one.

Blood flow

Another study examined alterations in muscle blood volume (Kerschan-Schindl et al 2001) with power Doppler sonography of the arterial blood flow of the popliteal artery. Twenty healthy adults stood with both feet on a tilting platform in three different positions for 3 min each without breaks in between. The amplitude was 3 mm and the frequency 26 Hz. The result of the study demonstrated an increase in mean blood flow velocity in the popliteal artery from 6.5 to 13.0 cm/s. Other investigators have demonstrated enhanced peripheral and systemic blood flow (25–35%), with improved lymphatic flow and better venous drainage (Stewart et al 2004). This suggests that low-frequency vibration does not have the same negative effects on peripheral circulation as seen in occupations with exposure to prolonged low-frequency vibration.

Proprioception and low back pain

In a pilot study by Fontana et al (2005) the effect of weight-bearing exercise in conjunction with low-frequency WBV was investigated to determine whether this combination would improve lumbosacral position sense in healthy subjects. Since patients with low back pain (LBP) often present with impaired proprioception of the lumbopelvic region (motor control dysfunction), which contributes to neuromuscular dysfunction and thereby impaired segmental stability (O'Sullivan et al 2003), the use of WBV may provide a useful treatment tool. Twenty-five individuals (eight men and 17 women) between the ages of 19 and 21 were randomly assigned to the experimental group ($n = 14$) and to the control group ($n = 11$). The experimental group received WBV using Galileo for 5 min with a frequency of 18 Hz and an amplitude of 10 mm (feet were placed apart). For the entire time the participants had to maintain a static semi-squat position during the WBV. The control group adopted the same position for an equal time but without receiving any vibration. A two-dimensional motion analysis system measured the repositioning accuracy of the pelvic tilt in standing was used. The results demonstrated that 5 min of WBV induced a decrease in absolute mean repositioning error, improving repositioning accuracy by 39% or 0.78°. Moreover, this was not dependent on the anterior or posterior repositioning of the pelvis. The net proportional benefit of the experimental group over the control group after the test was 53%. It was therefore concluded that WBVT has an effect on lumbosacral proprioception which had not been assessed in previous studies. Furthermore, this effect occurred with such a small amount of WBVT. These authors also stated that these results could provide a possible explanation for the beneficial findings by Rittweger et al (2002a) in their 12-week treatment programme in which they found an improvement in function and a relief in pain in patients with LBP. Further explanations for improved proprioception were also provided by Belavý et al (2008), who found that 8 weeks of WBV stimulated lumbar multifidus function. Atrophy of the multifidus muscle and loss of its proprioceptive function has been shown to be a significant contributor to chronic LBP (Hides 1996, Hodges 2004). Finally, Di Loreto et al (2004) found that WBV increased plasma norepinephrine concentrations (60 min: vibration 1.29 ± 0.18, control 1.01 ± 0.07 nM, $p = 0.038$). Direct descending noradrenergic pathways in the spinal cord have profound forward modulating effects on pain; however, the blood–brain barrier precludes plasma norepinephrine passing into the spinal cord. An indirect pathway for the resolution of pain may occur through the immune-inflammatory response as peripheral noradrenergic receptors innervate the blood vessels of the spleen, bones, nerves and lymphatic system.

Parkinson's disease

Vibration training has also been used to improve the symptoms of Parkinson's disease. Haas and colleagues (2006) have shown that 68 patients (15 women and 53 men) using WBVT have experienced improvements in one or more symptoms. A crossover design was used to control treatment effects on motor symptoms, which were assessed by the Unified Parkinson's Disease Rating Scale (UPDRS) motor score (Fig. 4.1). The treatment consisted of five sets of WBV lasting 60 s each with a 1-min pause between each series. The mean frequency of the vibration adopted was 6 Hz and the amplitude was 3 mm. In the treatment group, an improvement of 16.8% in the UPDRS motor score was found. The highest improvements were found in tremor and rigidity, 25 and 24%, respectively. Gait and posture showed an improvement of 15%, and bradykinesia scores were reduced by 12 on average, but no changes were found in cranial symptoms. It is worth emphasizing that these improvements were seen immediately after the intervention and lasted for 120 min, when the UPDRS score still had not returned to baseline. Moreover, correlation of the UPDRS with other functional psychometric questionaires and functional tests suggest that this is the strongest evidence yet for a (CNS) role in low-frequency WBV (Table 4.1).

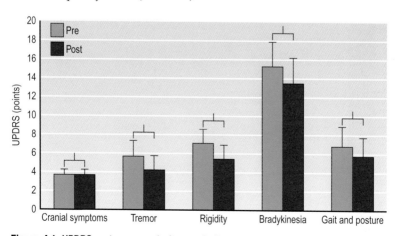

Figure 4.1 UPDRS motor scores before and after treatment in a five-symptom cluster.

Reprinted from Haas CT, Turbanski S, Kessler K et al (2006) The effects of random whole-body-vibration on motor symptoms in Parkinson's disease. *Neurological Rehabilitation* 21:29–36, with permission

Table 4.1 Comparisons between SF-36 psychometric scale, functional capacity evaluation and UPDRS

Test performed	n	Mean (SD)[a]	95% CI[a]	ICC[D]	MDC[95]
Balance tests					
Berg Balance Scale (0–56 points)	37	50 (7)	47–52	0.94	5
Activities-specific Balance Confidence Scale (%)	36	70 (19)	64–77	0.94	13
Functional Reach Test (cm)					
Forward	37	21 (6)	18–23	0.73	9
Backward	36	14 (5)	13–16	0.67	7
Romberg Test (s)					
Eyes open	37	58 (10)	55–62	0.86	10
Eyes closed	37	54 (17)	48–60	0.84	19
Sharpened Romberg Test (s)					
Eyes open	37	39 (25)	30–47	0.70	39
Eyes closed	37	15 (22)	8–23	0.91	19
Ambulation tests					
Six-Minute Walk Test (m)	37	316 (142)	269–364	0.96	82
Timed 'Up & Go' Test (s)	37	15 (10)	12–19	0.85	11

	N	Mean (SD)	95% CI	ICC	
gait speed (m/s)					
Comfortable	36	1.16 (.34)	1.04–1.27	0.96	0.18
Fast	36	1.47 (.51)	1.30–1.64	0.97	0.25
36-Item Short-Form Health Survey (0–100 points)					
Physical functioning	36	57 (23)	49–65	0.80	28
Role-physical	36	47 (41)	33–61	0.85	45
Bodily pain	36	68 (27)	59–77	0.89	25
General health	36	59 (26)	50–67	0.85	28
Vitality	36	52 (20)	45–59	0.88	19
Social functioning	36	83 (20)	76–90	0.71	29
Role-emotional	36	75 (40)	61–89	0.84	45
Mental health	36	76 (16)	70–81	0.83	19
Unified Parkinson Disease Rating Scale (points)					
Mentation, behaviour, and mood (0–16)	36	2 (2)	2–3	0.89	2
Activities of daily living (0–52)	36	12 (6)	10–14	0.93	4
Motor examination (0–108)	37	19 (12)	15–23	0.89	11
Total score (0–176)	36	33 (16)	28–38	0.91	13

[a] Means, standard deviations, and 95% confidence intervals (CIs) are from the first day of testing.

[b] ICC (3,1): Berg Balance Scale, Activities-specific Balance Confidence Scale, Romberg Test, Sharpened Romberg Test, Six-Minutes Walk Test, 36-Item Short-Form Health Survey, and Unified Parkinson Disease Rating Scale. ICC (3,2): Functional Reach Test, Timed 'Up & Go' Test, and gait speed.

Reprinted from Steffen T, Seney M (2008) Test-retest reliability and minimal detectable change on balance and ambulation tests, the 36-tiem short-form healthy survey, and the unified Parkinson disease rating scale in people with parkinsonism. Physical Therapy 88(6):733–746.

Stroke

van Nes et al (2004) indicated that WBV may have a positive impact on postural proprioception in people suffering from stroke. Balance was assessed in 23 patients with unilateral chronic stroke over four trials. The participants in this study were asked to stand quietly on a dual plate force platform (this unit has two vibrating plates, allowing the user to place one foot on each plate), with open and closed eyes while performing a voluntary weight-shifting task. The four trials were carried out at 45-min intervals, and between the second and the third assessment, four repetitions of 45 s of vibration with a frequency of 30 Hz and an amplitude of 3 mm were given. The results demonstrated an improvement in weight-shifting speed while maintaining the precision of movement.

Multiple sclerosis

WBV was used in 12 people with moderate disability as a result of multiple sclerosis (MS). A frequency of 2–4.4 Hz, with an amplitude of 3 mm, in five series of 1-min stimulation with a 1-min break was used in a randomized control study. In comparison with the placebo group the treatment group demonstrated improvements in sensory organization tests and the timed get up and go (GUG) test with a pre-application score of 9.2 s, whereas the post-application score was 8.2 s up to 1 week after the application of WBV. The mean values of the posturographic scores were 70.5 before application and 77.5 1 week after the WBV. No differences were found in the functional reach test.

Conclusions of acute effects

The acute effects described above are an indication as to the initial frequency of WBV required for sporting endeavours and various therapeutic interventions. More importantly, these results allow the possibility of immediately measuring the response to WBV. Furthermore, by measuring responses to WBV it gives the clinician a valid reason for continuing, discontinuing, changing or progressing treatment. Changing or progressing treatment would be based on the predictive reasoning of expected outcomes. As expectations of the predictive reasoning are met, the clinical validity of this approach can be justified to the client, insurers and health organizations. In turn it can provide researchers with a stimulus for future investigations in which the clinical parameters become more tightly defined for various populations.

A barrage of outcome measures for impairment and disability or for sporting achievement have been described. Importantly by using impairment and functional scales the minimum criteria for validity is being met. The few centimetre improvements in jump height or the minimum improvement in CMJ should reflect changes in dynamic quadriceps and calf power, as well as improvements in athletic achievements for concurrent validity to be established. Naturally, other variables outside of the clinician's practice may also be involved; yet minimal detectable improvements may result in the ultimate outcome of highest sporting achievement. Similarly, at the other end of the spectrum, the elderly institutionalized clients who may even be bed-ridden and require a tilt table for the application of WBV also have outcomes to be measured which reflect the ultimate goal of re-ambulation. These may commence with their physiological response to standing, their ability to stand (GUG test) balance [activities-specific balance confidence (ABC), Falls Efficacy Scale (FES), Tinnetti balance tool, Berg Balance Scale] and finally walking (six minute Walk Test or derivations thereof). Hopefully, the clinician then finds that these functional improvements are reflected on the SF-36, where WBV has been shown to improve the items in physical function, pain, vitality and general health (Bruyere et al 2005). In this manner incremental & concurrent validity is achieved, since these tests have been demonstrated to be valid and reliable. Although WBV has had only limited RCTs to justify its use, the clinician's outcomes should be rigorous enough to justify further treatment funding. In this way the cart isn't placed before the horse and the general public does not have to wait for the research to justify the means.

To summarize, the frequency for muscle relaxation should be <20 Hz. To improve parameters regarding muscle strength, frequencies between 26 and 44 Hz are used in the lower limbs, and up to 50 Hz when using dumbbells. Frequencies above 50 Hz will probably cause muscle damage and therefore should be avoided. The parameter of amplitude remains largely undefined; however, the range is 1–10 mm and it would appear that the greater the amplitude, the greater the fatigue of the calf muscles. The duration of WBV ranges from 1 to 10 min. With longer durations and high intensity, at least one 6-min rest period should be instigated for athletes. With the frail and deconditioned, the 3×1-min protocol of small amplitude with 60 s rest between each repetition appears to be a prudent starting point. Variation from static to dynamic posture with various levels of squatting as well as one-legged balance and movement have been proposed for progression.

Long-term effects of WBV using the variables of duration, frequency, body positioning and amplitude

Fortunately, investigations into the long-term effects of WBV seem to provide more supportive evidence in a wide range of subjects including athletes, active people, sedentary people and older populations. Using WBVT over a period of time appears to have the potential to elicit a long-term training effect on muscle strength and functional performance, power, motor control, balance, chronic pain and bone density (Bosco et al

1998, Issurin et al 1994, Judex et al 2007, Mester et al 1999, Rittweger et al 2002a, Rubin et al 2001, 2004, 2007, Runge et al 2000, Torvinen et al 2002b, Xie et al 2006). Furthermore, investigations into the long-term effect of WBVT can provide us with further insights into the dosage of training in regard to duration and frequency (the number of times per week), as well as suggesting guidelines for effective progression of training. This latter aspect is of particular importance as it not only frames an issue of safety but similar to progressive resistance training, as has been advocated by the American College of Sports Medicine (ACSM), progression of exercise prescription is a cornerstone for the treatment of morbidity associated with inactivity and metabolic syndrome.

Variable methods of dosage for progression

Rittweger et al (2000, 2001, 2002a,b, 2003) demonstrated several methods of dosage for progressive training. In Rittweger et al (2000) they used 26 Hz, feet 15 cm from rotation axis, vibration amplitude 1.05 cm, peak acceleration 147 m/s^2 = 15g with squatting + additional load 40% body weight, 3 s down, 3 s up to elicit a physiological fatiguing response. In 2001 they used 26 Hz, 6 mm, amplitude feet 24 cm apart (approx. 18g based on 30 Hz) with 3 min squatting in cycles of 6 s, simple standing, squatting with an additional 35% body weight load for females and 40% load for males to elicit increased oxygen consumption. In Rittweger et al (2002a) they used 18 Hz, 6 mm, 4 min initially, gradually increased to 7 min in which 18 exercise units were performed within 12 weeks, with two units in the first 6 weeks and then one unit per week thereafter, on a Galileo 2000, in static slight knee flexion, bending in the frontal and sagittal plane and rotating in the horizontal plane; 5 kg was added to the shoulders in later sessions to treat LBP. In Rittweger et al (2000b) they used 18–34 Hz, 5 mm, with the addition of 40% lean body mass attached to waist and later shoulders; whereas in Rittweger et al (2003) they used 26 Hz (used because below 20 Hz induces relaxation, whereas above 50 Hz can induce severe muscle damage), 6 mm (12 mm from top to bottom) with a Galileo 2000 prototype, 0–90° knee flexion, plus 40% lean body mass added to the hips, 3 s down and 3 s up, exercise until exhaustion to test CNS contributions to fatigue. Similarly, Bosco et al (1999b) used heavy loading in physically active people. Their protocol included 26 Hz, amplitude 10 mm, acceleration 27 m/s^2, standing on toes, half, squat, feet rotated externally, single right leg 90° squat, single left leg 90° squat (with the last two positions subjects could maintain balance using a bar) with vertical sinusoidal vibrations lasting 90 s each, with 40 s break between sets for a total of 10 min/day; every day, 5 s was added until 2 min per position was reached. These authors calculated that this cumulative load of WBV of 100 min at 2.7g was equivalent to the intensity of 200 drop jumps from 60 cm twice a week for 12 months (moreover, the total time for a drop jump is only 200 ms and the acceleration developed cannot reach 2.7g). Furthermore, using a Gallileo 2000, at 26 Hz, 10 mm, acceleration = 54 m/s^2 with WBV and one leg in 100° flexion, 10 times for 60 s each, with 60 s rest in between. Total time was 10 min WBV at 5.4g = 150 leg presses or half-squats with extra loads (three times body weight), twice per week for 5 weeks. Together, these investigations demonstrate variable parameters which can be used for adaptability of training protocols depending upon the population in which they are being used and the outcome which the subjects wish to achieve. This makes perfect clinical sense. Importantly, this latter research makes direct calculable comparisons of WBV with other forms of plyometric exercise.

The long-term effects of progression on outcome measures

Outcome measures such as jumping and CMJ have been used extensively to assess the effect of WBV. Investigators found that 10 days of WBV training resulted in an increase in average jumping height (+11.9%) and power output during repeated hopping in active subjects, but no change in CMJ performance. The parameters used during the procedure were a frequency of 26 Hz with a 10-mm displacement for a total time of exposure of 100 min (Bosco et al 1998). In a randomized controlled study conducted over a 4-month period, WBVT was performed with static and dynamic squatting exercises, and was shown to induce an 8.5% net improvement in the jumping height in 56 young healthy non-athletic volunteers. Lower limb extension strength increased after 2 months of vibration intervention, resulting in 3.7% enhancement. However, this improvement slowed down by the end of the intervention and, after 4 months, the difference between the vibration group and the control group was no longer statistically significant. This may have been due to the learning effect, whereby the control group increased the extension strength. Parameters utilized in the present study were platform vibration amplitude 2 mm where the frequency ranged between 25 and 40 Hz and the acceleration force ranged between 2.5 and 6.4g. Interestingly, concepts of progression were utilized here in which, for the first 2 weeks, 25 Hz for 1 min was used then 30 Hz for another minute was applied. For the next 1.5 months, it was 3 min of 25 Hz/60 s + 30 Hz/60 s + 35 Hz/60 s, and then for the remaining 2 months, 4 min of 25 Hz/60 s + 30 Hz/60 s + 35 Hz/60 s + 40 Hz/60 s. Acceleration was 2.5g at 25 Hz, 3.6g at 30 Hz, 4.9g at 35 Hz and 6.4g at 40 Hz. Duration, frequency and type of exercise include 4 min/day 3–5 times per week, 4 × 60 s, light squatting (0–10 s), standing in the erect position (10–20 s), standing relaxed knees slightly flexed (20–30 s), light jumping (30–40 s), alternating the body weight from one leg to the other (40–50 s), standing on the heels (50–60 s) (Torvinen et al 2002b). It is interesting to note that no further improvement occurred after 2 months, which coincides with the slowing of progression.

In a placebo-controlled study investigators reported enhancement in isometric, dynamic and explosive strength (power) of knee extensor muscles in 67 untrained young healthy women (21.4 ± 1.8 years) following 12 weeks of WBV training (Delecluse et al 2003). Participants were placed into four different groups: WBV (WBV, n = 18), a placebo group (PL, n = 19), a resistance-training group (RES, n = 18), and a control group (n = 12). The WBV and the PL groups performed static and dynamic knee-extensor exercises (squats, deep squats, wide-stance squats, one-legged squats and lunges) on a vibration platform three times per week. In the WBV group the platform had a frequency of 35–40 Hz and the amplitude was 2.5–5 mm. Over the 12 weeks, the WBV group went from 3-min training per session to 20 min, increasing the number of repetitions per exercise, shortening the rest periods or increasing the frequency and/or the amplitude of the vibration. The PL group performed the same exercise standing on the platform, could hear the noise (motor) and felt tingles in their feet, but the acceleration of the platform was only 0.4g with negligible amplitude. The RES group performed a moderate resistance training programme for knee extensor on a leg press and leg extension machine. The resistance training programme was slowly progressive, similar to the WBV programme. The results showed that isometric and dynamic knee extensor strength increased significantly in both the WBV group (16.6 and 9% respectively) and the RES group (14.4 and 7% respectively), whereas the PL and control group did not show any significant increase. Additionally, the CMJ height enhanced significantly (7.6%) only in the WBV group. Clearly, the findings suggest that WBV, and the reflexive muscle contraction it provokes, has the potential to induce strength gain in knee extensor in a group of untrained women and may be just as effective as resistance training at moderate intensity (Vella 2005). These authors concluded that the strength enhancement that resulting from WBVT were not attributable to a placebo effect (Delecluse et al 2003). However, it should be noted that in the present study the resistance exercise programme (leg press and leg extension) was performed to failure without explosive movements, thereby reducing the possibility of producing significant changes in explosive measures.

In a similar study, the same researchers reported a significant increase in fat-free mass and in the force–velocity relation of knee extensor muscles in untrained female subjects. This study compared the effects of WBV, using a frequency of 35–40 Hz and an amplitude of 2.5–5 mm, with resistance training over a period of 24 weeks on body composition and knee extensor strength. No significant changes were seen in body weight or percentage of body fat in either group. However, the WBV group demonstrated a significant increase in fat-free mass (2.2%), whereas increases in knee extensor strength were reported in both groups (Roelants et al 2004b). In another study conducted by Roelants et al (2004a) a 24-week programme of WBV training performed three times per week increased dynamic knee extensor strength in postmenopausal women by 15%. This result was similar to the result reported in the resistance trained group. The WBV group demonstrated, in contrast to the resistance trained group, an enhancement in the speed of movement of the knee extensors, supporting the concept that WBV may be superior to resistance training for increasing power as a large determinant of muscular power is speed of movement. Progression was achieved through the use of 35–40 Hz, 2.5–5.0 mm using a Power Plate with a total duration of 5 to 30 min by the end of training.

Bone mineral density (BMD) and muscle strength

Common to all these studies was that the standard training groups were not significantly different from each other and therefore one can observe that the results demonstrate that long-term programmes of WBV training can produce significant improvements in leg extensor muscle strength in an untrained female population. Another supporting study was published by the same group of people (Verschueren et al 2004). Seventy volunteers (age, 58–74 years) were randomly assigned to a WBV group, a resistance training group (RES) or a control group (CON). The WBV and the RES groups trained three times per week for a period of 6 months. The WBV group performed static and dynamic knee extensor exercises on a vibration platform (35–40 Hz, 2.28–5.09g). The RES group trained knee extensors by dynamic leg press and leg extension exercises, increasing from low to high resistance. The CON group did not participate in any training. No vibration-related side-effects were observed in these participants. The results demonstrated that the WBV group improved isometric and dynamic muscle strength (+15 and +16%, respectively) and was also determined to be effective for increasing BMD of the hip even though the improvement was very small (+0.93%) but within the error of measurement used for establishing BMD. No changes in hip BMD were observed in women participating in the RES group.

Similar results were found by Gusi et al (2006) whereby BMD of the femoral neck increased by 4.3% more in the WBV-trained people than in their control walking group. BMD of the lumbar spine was unaltered in both groups. Balance improved in the WBV group by 29%. Their programme consisted of three sessions per week for 8 months, for six bouts of 1 min (12.6 Hz, 3-cm amplitude, 60° knee flexion). Prevention of postmenopausal bone loss using WBV was demonstrated by Rubin et al (2004). They used two 10-min treatments per day of 30 Hz vertical acceleration at 2 m/s² peak-to-peak acceleration for 12 months. The placebo subjects lost 2.13% in the femoral neck over 1 year, whereas the WBV group gained 0.04% (net benefit of 2.17%). In the spine, the placebo group lost 1.6% over the year, where as the WBV group only lost 0.10%. Taken together, this is very encouraging evidence for the use of WBV in postmenopausal women.

De Ruiter et al (2003b) analysed the effects of 11 weeks of WBV at 30 Hz and 8-mm amplitude training on maximal voluntary contraction, maximal force-generating capacity and electrically stimulated maximal rate of force rise. The subjects had WBVT three times per week starting with five sets of 1 min, increasing up to eight sets of 1 min each. After every set there was a 1-min rest and between week 5 and week 7 there was a cessation of training for 2 weeks. Although the total exposure time on WBVT was 169 min, the results showed no change in all parameters tested except for an increase in electrically stimulated maximal rate of force rise. However, their training protocols were not progressive and therefore violate the essence of training principles. Nevertheless, these investigations clearly demonstrate that, if WBVT is performed with physically active people for a short period of time and with small amplitude, there will not be a big change or improvement in power-generating capacity of the lower limb. Again the overloading principle of training regimen has been ignored. Therefore, if the aim of vibration exercise is to enhance neuromuscular performance, one must be aware that, in well-trained people, an optimal amplitude and frequency should be coupled with an optimal level of muscle activity on which the vibration stimulation can be superimposed (Cardinale & Wakeling 2005). Since good results were achieved when progressive loading was used in sedentary individuals (Delecluse et al 2003, Torvinen et al 2002b), the rule of progressive overloading must be applied at the appropriate level in the population being investigated. Clinically this is intuitive practice based on observable outcome measures. Future investigation should address progressive loading and normative starting points in various populations.

Improvements in proprioception, muscle hypertrophy, motor control and bone density for the treatment of low back pain

A series of studies by Lundeberg et al (1984) demonstrated that relatively low-frequency vibration also reduced pain. In contrast, occupational WBV produced by heavy machinery and pneumatic hammers has been viewed as a risk factor for chronic LBP (Skovron 1992). In these instances, workers have been exposed to vibration for long durations or to large magnitudes of vibration for a short period of time. Examples include jack-leg-type drills in miners in whom the total exposure to vibration is up to 3 hours per day. Clearly, in these cases, the body passively absorbed vibration, over a long period of time, with the potential for damaging musculoskeletal and neural structures. The low-frequency, short duration, focused exercise programmes of WBV differ markedly from those of occupational hazards. In fact, therapeutic WBV may be part of the cure rather than the cause of LBP (Rittweger et al 2002a).

Rittweger et al (2002a) compared the effects of WBV and isometric exercises on lumbar strength, pain and disability rating in 60 female and male patients (mean age of 51.7 years) with chronic LBP (mean history of 13.1 years). In this RCT, subjects performed either isodynamic lumbar extension exercise (LEX) or vibration exercise for 3 months. In both groups, two exercise units per week were performed for the first 6 weeks and then only one unit per week thereafter. The people using WBV exercised on a Galileo platform with an amplitude of 6 mm and a vibration frequency of 18 Hz for a period of 4–7 min. During the exercise units, the participant was asked to perform slow movements of the hips and waist, with bending in different planes and rotation in the transverse plane. Outcome measures of this study were lumbar extension torque, pain sensation (visual analogue scale) and pain-related disability (pain disability index). Results demonstrated significant and comparable reductions in pain sensation ($p < 0.001$) and pain-related disability ($p < 0.01$) in both groups. Lumbar extension torque increased significantly more in the lumbar extension group ($p < 0.05$) than in the vibration exercise group. Interestingly, no correlation was found between gain in lumbar torque and pain relief or pain-related disability ($p < 0.2$). Therefore, WBVT exercise seems to be a valid form of treatment for people with chronic LBP.

In a 12-month trial, 48 young women with a history of at least one skeletal fracture and low BMD underwent 10 min of WBV at 30 Hz and 0.3g. The results demonstrated marked improvements in BMD of the femoral mid-shaft cortical bone by 2.1% and lumbar vertebrae cancellous bone by 3.4%. Generally greater improvements by 2.0 and 2.3% in the cancellous and trabecular bones were seen in the WBV group (Table 4.2). Moreover, muscle hypertrophy was demonstrated.

The effects of vibration on pain relief may be mediated through its effects on motor control, especially on the function of the antigravity muscle system. Issurin and Tenenbaum (1999) stated that, when vibration is applied from distal to proximal, an optimal effect occurs on muscle activation and recruitment patterns of the antigravity, weight-bearing muscles. This means that a specific WBV training would have a positive effect on patients with LBP, based on the direct effect on increasing sensory input (proprioceptive) to the local and weight-bearing muscles. People with LBP often present with impaired proprioception at the lumbopelvic region. Therefore, in order to treat them effectively, proprioceptive train-

Table 4.2 Improvements in muscle cross-sectional area and bone density in 'high compliers' undergoing WBV

	Absolute change			Percentage change		
	Control + poor compliers	High compliers	p	Control + poor compliers	High compliers	p
Axial						
Total paraspinous musculature (cm²)	1.4 ± 8.9	12.6 ± 12.6	0.001	0.8 ± 5.1	8.0 ± 9.1	0.001
Psoas (cm²)	0.6 ± 3.6	3.1 ± 2.8	0.01	1.6 ± 8.2	6.8 ± 6.0	0.02
Quadratus lumborum (cm²)	1.1 ± 2.5	2.4 ± 2.7	0.11	5.4 ± 13.7	13.4 ± 15.0	0.07
Erector spinae (cm²)	−0.3 ± 5.3	7.1 ± 10.4	0.002	−0.2 ± 4.7	8.1 ± 14.5	0.006
Spine cancellous BMD (mg/cm³)	−0.4 ± 7.4	5.9 ± 7.2	0.006	−0.1 ± 4.5	3.8 ± 4.9	0.007
Appendicular						
Quadriceps femoris area (cm²)	3.0 ± 7.8	4.0 ± 4.5	0.59	3.0 ± 6.8	3.9 ± 4.2	0.63
Femur cross-sectional area (cm²)	0.05 ± 0.12	0.12 ± 0.16	0.10	1.0 ± 2.2	2.4 ± 3.7	0.12
Femur cortical bone area (cm²)	0.05 ± 0.17	0.17 ± 0.13	0.02	1.3 ± 3.9	4.3 ± 3.6	0.009

Highly significant differences were observed in several regions of the spine musculature, as well as the cancellous bone of the spine and cortical bone area of the hip, whereas musculature around the femur and cross-sectional area of the femur were not significantly different between groups.
Reproduced from Gilsanz V, Wren TAL, Sanchez M et al (2006) Low-level high frequency mechanical signals enhance musculoskeletal development of young women with low. BMD. *Journal of Bone and Mineral Research* 21(9):1464–1474, with permission from the American Society for Bone and Mineral Research.

ing becomes an important part of the rehabilitation programme. In cases with unilateral loss of muscle function it may be possible that the alternating oscillatory movement provides a comparative input to the CNS which then can adjust its muscle tone and hence afferent firing appropriate for balance between the two sides of the body. Evidence for such a hypothesis comes from researchers who found that 5 min of 18-Hz WBV induced a decrease in absolute mean repositioning error, in healthy subjects (Fontana et al 2005). Since proprioception improved, one can hypothesize that people with LBP should profit from this result. This finding provides a possible explanation as to why other investigators found an improvement in function and a relief in LBP after a 12-week programme of WBV (Rittweger et al 2002a). The multifidus muscle has been shown to be frequently atrophied in people with LBP and this was considered to reduce the proprioceptive capacity in the spine (Hides et al 1996). WBV has been shown to prevent the atrophying effects of bed rest on the multifidus muscle as well as prevent morphological compensatory changes in the erector spinae muscles (Belavý et al 2008). Additionally, weakness of the pelvic floor has been implicated in altered activation of the deep abdominal muscles and LBP (Sapsford et al 2005). Von der Heide et al (2004) found that WBV in combination with physiotherapy improved the subjective and objective parameters of stress urinary incontinence. This thereby provides further indirect evidence for the potential pain-relieving effect of WBV.

Pantaleo et al (1986) showed that vibration at 110 Hz resulted in a reduction in pain sensation, whereas vibration at 30 Hz failed to reduce pain sensations. They investigated the effects of vibratory stimulation on muscular pain threshold of the vastus medialis muscle in 28 healthy subjects. In all the subjects tested, high-frequency vibration (110 Hz) induced a marked and long-lasting elevation of the muscular pain threshold but only when vibration was applied to the skin overlying the ipsilateral quadriceps tendon or neighbouring areas and not when applied to remote ipsi- or contralateral regions. Stimulation of vibration at 30 Hz failed to produce any effect on muscular pain threshold. However, a facilitation of the blink response, not accompanied by changes in pain sensation, was observed during the first period of both high- and low-frequency vibratory stimulation. The authors concluded the study explains how vibration would be able to affect pain sensation. They suggested a role for rapidly adapting receptors and/or pacinian corpuscles in this effect and support the hypothesis of an inhibition of nociceptive messages, possibly at spinal segmental levels, by volleys in large myelinated afferent fibres.

Inability to make minor muscular adjustments to posture, in people with LBP has been thought to be symptomatic of excessive muscular splinting around the spine (Hodges 2004). Such motor control issues could be driven from higher centres of the central nervous system. Evidence for improved CNS motor control after WBV comes from investigations into neurological conditions. Improvements in balance were found when four trials of WBV were applied to 23 patients suffering from the effects of unilateral chronic stroke (van Nes et al 2004). One can hypothesize that improvements in motor control were partially responsible for this effect. Indeed, evidence from investigations into Parkinson's disease has shown that WBVT can improve symptoms such as tremor, rigidity, balance and postural stability. In their research, Haas et al (2006) could demonstrate that 3–5 sets of 45–60 s (with 30–60 s recovery) vibration at a frequency of 4–7 Hz would improve Parkinson's symptoms, which was seen as quickly as 10–60 min after the intervention and lasted for 2–48 hours. This appears to have been from a CNS effect on muscle relaxation. When one considers that many painful conditions are associated with reflexogenic muscle spasms and excessive 'force closure' around joints (O'Sullivan et al 2003) then WBV may be postulated to relieve some of these compressive forces through muscle relaxation.

A form of WBV has been used to enhance the effects of end of range stretching in gymnastics. It was postulated that a phenomenon of pain alleviation or a shift in pain threshold contributed to the positive effect of WBVT through a reduction in pain and therefore greater temptation to stretch further (Issurin & Tenenbaum 1999, Sands et al 2006). Since painful stimuli from stretching are common in those sports that involve serious stretching and extreme ranges of motion, a reduction in pain might allow the subject to proceed to greater ranges of motion before pain inhibits progress. Generally speaking the aim of many training regimen is to optimize biomechanical parameters and thereby maximize performance and minimize the risk of injury. Therefore, the enhanced ranges of motion (Kinser et al 2008, Sands et al 2006, Van den Tillaar 2006) and improvements in strength (Bosco et al 1999a) described in the literature suggest that WBV could also be seen as pain preventive.

Vibration training exercise appears to improve functional capacity and vitality in the elderly. Improvements in physical function and psycho-cognitive domain items in the SF-36 scale have been demonstrated after 6 weeks of WBV (Bruyere et al 2005) (Fig. 4.2). Therefore, indirect effects on pain through enhanced independence in nursing home clients can be considered a consequence of WBV.

Currently, WBV can be seen as a tool in the multidimensional and hence multimodal approach to treating pain. At present, the direct role of WBV on pain receptors in joints and muscles is unknown. Furthermore, the effect on the sympathetic and immune systems still needs to be ascertained. Nevertheless, in the absence of contraindications, WBV is likely to be found to be beneficial if applied in a dose-specific manner.

SF-36® Scales measure physical and mental components of health

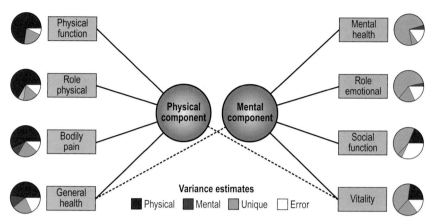

Figure 4.2 SF-36 scale. Reprinted from Ware JE, Kosinski M, & Keller SD. SF-36 Physical and Mental Health Summary Scales: A User Manual. Boston, MA: Health Assessment Lab, 1994, with permission.

Elderly and function

Bogaerts and collegues (2006) conducted a randomized controlled study investigating the effects of 1-year WBVT on isometric and explosive muscle strength and muscle mass in community-dwelling men older than 60 years. Kawanabe et al (2007) used 12–20 Hz WBV for 4 min, once per week for 2 months. They found walking speed (–14.9%), step length (+6.5%), and maximum standing time on one leg (right +65%, left +88.4%) improved significantly in the WBV plus exercise group. Moreover, no serious adverse events occurred during the study period.

Conclusion

These investigations demonstrate varying results. All of these investigations are applicable clinically for determining appropriate outcome measures. Some of the investigations demonstrate the need for progressive training due to their poor results while others highlight how progressive loading can be attained. Although various populations which may benefit from WBV have been defined, there appear to be subpopulations which appear to benefit more from WBV than others. Moreover, these investigations have identified parameters and variables of safety as well as logical progression. Importantly, the clinician has been presented with a barrage of evaluation techniques which can be used not only to establish efficacy of treatment but also to determine the stage at which progression is appropriate and/or when treatment should cease. It would appear that WBV may integrate well with other functional forms of exercise. Interested readers should refer to the Appendix for summaries of these investigations as well as information on evaluation.

References

Abercromby AFJ, Amonette WE, Layne CS, Mcfarlin BK, Hinman MR, Paloski WH (2007a) Variation in neuromuscular responses during acute whole-body vibration exercise. *Medicine and Science in Sport and Exercise* 1642–1650.

Abercromby AFJ, Amonette WE, Layne CS Mcfarlin BK, Hinman MR, Paloski WH (2007b) Vibration exposure and biodynamic responses during whole-body vibration training. *Medicine and Science in Sport and Exercise* 1794–1800.

Bautmans I, Van Hees E, Lemper J-L et al (2005) The feasibility of whole body vibration in institutionalised elderly persons and its influence on muscle performance, balance and mobility: a randomised controlled trial. *BMC Geriatrics* 5:17.

Belavý DL, Hides JA, Wilson SJ et al (2008) Resistive simulated weight bearing exercise with whole body vibration reduces lumbar spine deconditioning in bed-rest. *Spine* 33(5):121–131.

Bogaerts An, Verschueren S, Delecluse C et al (2006) Impac of whole body vibration training versus fitness training on muscle strength and muscle mass in older men: a 1 year randomized controlled trial. *Journal of Gerontology* 62A(6):630–635.

Bosco C, Cardinale M, Tsarpela O (1998) The influence of vibration of whole-body vibrations on jumping performance. *Biology of Sports* 15:157–164.

Bosco C, Cardinale M, Tsarpela O (1999) Influence of vibration on mechanical power and electromyogram activity in human arm flexor muscles. *European Journal of Applied Physiology* 79:306–311.

Bosco C, Colli R, Introini E et al (1999a) Adaptive responses of human skeletal muscle to vibration exposure. *Clinical Physiology* 19(2):183–187.

Bosco C, Cardinale M, Tsarpela O (1999b) Influence of vibration on mechanical power and electromyogram activity in human arm flexor muscles. *European Journal of Applied Physiology* 79:306–311.

Bosco C, Iacovelli M, Tsarpela O et al (2000) Hormonal responses to whole-body vibration in men. *European Journal of Applied Physiolology* 81(6):449–454.

Bruyere O, Wuidart MA, Di Palma E et al (2005) Controlled whole body vibration to decrease fall risk and improve health-related quality of life of nursing home residents. *Archives of Physical Medicine and Rehabilitation* 86:303–307.

Cardinale M (2002) The effects of vibration on human performance and hormonal profile. Doctoral thesis, Semmelweis University, Hungary.

Cardinale M, Wakeling J (2005) Whole body vibration exercise: are vibrations good for you? *British Journal of Sports Medicine* 39: 585–589.

Cochrane DJ, Stannard SR, Walmsley A et al (2007) The acute effect of vibration exercise on concentric muscular characteristic. *Journal of Science and Medicine in Sport* 11(6):527–534.

Delecluse C, Roelants M, Verschueren S (2003) Strength increase after whole-body vibration compared with resistance training. *Medicine and Science in Sports and Exercise* 35(6):1033–1041.

De Ruiter CJ, van der Linden RM, van der Zijden MJ et al (2003a) Short-term effects of whole-body vibration on maximal voluntary isometric knee extensor force and rate of force rise. *European Journal of Applied Physiology* 88:472–475.

De Ruiter CJ, Van Raak SM, Schilperoort JV et al (2003b) The effects of 11 weeks whole body vibration training on jump height contractile properties and activation of human knee extensors. *European Journal of Applied Physiology* 90:595–600.

Di Loreto C, Ranchelli A, Lucidi P et al (2004) Effects of whole-body vibration exercise on the endocrine system of healthy men. *Journal of Endocrinological Investigation* 27:323–327.

Eklund G (1972) Position sense and state of contraction: the effects of vibration. *Journal of Neurology, Neurosurgery and Psychiatry* 35:606–611.

Fontana TL, Richardson CA, Stanton WR (2005) The effect of weightbearing exercise with low frequency, whole body vibration on lumbosacral proprioception: A pilot study on normal subjects. *Australian Journal of Physiotherapy* 51:259–263.

Griffin MJ (1996) *Handbook of Human Vibration*. Academic Press, San Diego.

Gusi N, Raimundo A, Leal A (2006) Low frequency vibratory exercise reduces the risk of bone fracture more than walking: a randomized controlled trial. *BMC Musculoskeletal Disorders* 7:92.

Haas CT, Turbanski S, Kessler K et al (2006) The effects of random whole-body-vibration on motor symptoms in Parkinson's disease. *Neurological Rehabilitation* 21:29–36.

Hazell TJ, Jakobi JM, Kenno KA (2007) The effects of whole-body vibration on upper- and lower-body EMG during static and dynamic contractions. *Applied Physiology of Nutrition and Metabolism* 32(6):1156–1163.

Hides JA, Richardson CA, Jull GA (1996) Multifidus muscle recovery is not automatic after resolution of acute first-episode low back pain. *Spine* 21:2763–2769.

Hodges P (2004) Abdominal mechanism in low back pain. In: Richardson C, Hodges P, Hide J (eds) *Therapeutic Exercise for Lumbopelvic Stabilization: A Motor Control Approach for the Treatment and Prevention of Low Back Pain*, 2nd edn (Churchill Livingston, Edinburgh), pp 141–148.

Issurin V, Tenenbaum G (1999) Acute and residual effects of vibratory stimulation on explosive strength in elite and amateur athletes. *Journal of Sports Sciences* 17:177–182.

Issurin V, Liebermann DG, Tenenbaum G (1994) Effect of vibratory stimulation training on maximal force and flexibility. *Journal of Sports Sciences* 12:561–566.

Jordan JM, Norris SR, Smith DJ et al (2005) Vibration training: an overview of the area training consequences and future considerations. *Journal of Strength and Conditioning Research* 19(2):459–466.

Judex S, Lei X, Han D et al (2007) Low-magnitude mechanical signals that stimulate bone formation in the ovariectomized rat are dependent on the applied frequency but not on the strain magnitude. *Journal of Biomechanics* 40:1333–1339.

Kawanabe K, Kawashima A, Sashimoto I et al (2007) Effect of whole-body vibration exercise and muscle strengthening on walking ability in the elderly. *Keio Journal of Medicine* 56(1):28–33.

Kerschan-Schindl K, Gramp S, Henk C et al (2001) Whole-body vibration exercise leads to alterations in muscle blood volume. *Clinical Physiology* 21(3):377–382.

Kinser AM, Ramsey MW, O'Bryant HS et al (2008) Vibration and stretching effects on flexibility and explosive strength in young gymnasts. *Medicine and Science in Sports and Exercise* 40(1):133–140.

Kitazaki S, Griffin MJ (1997) A model analysis of whole body vertical vibration, using a finite element model of the human body. *Journal of Sound and Vibration* 200(1):83–103.

Lundeberg T, Nordemar R, Ottoson D (1984) Pain alleviation by vibratory stimulation. *Pain* 20:25–44.

Mester J, Spitzenfeil P, Schwarzer J et al (1999) Biological reaction to vibration: implication for sport. *Journal of Science and Medicine in Sport* 2:211–226.

Moran K, McNamara B, Luo J (2007) Effect of vibration training in maximal effort (70% 1RM) dynamic bicep curls. *Medicine and Science in Sports and Exercise* 39(3):526–533.

O'Sullivan PB, Burnett A, Floyd AN et al (2003) Lumbar repositioning deficit in a specific low back pain population *Spine* 28:1074–1079.

Pantaleo T, Duranti R, Bellini F (1986) Effects of vibratory stimulation on muscular pain threshold and blink response in human subjects. *Pain* 24:239–250.

Rittweger J, Beller G, Felsenberg D (2000) Acute physiological effects of exhaustive whole-body vibration exercise in man. *Clinical Physiology* 20:134–142.

Rittweger J, Schiessl H, Felsenberg D (2001) Oxygen uptake during whole-body vibration exercise: comparison with squatting as a slow voluntary movement. *European Journal of Applied Physiology* 86:169–173.

Rittweger J, Just K, Kautzsch K et al (2002a) Treatment of chronic lower back pain with lumbar extension and whole-body vibration exercise. *Spine* 27(17):1829–1834.

Rittweger J, Ehrig J, Just K et al (2002b) Oxygen uptake in whole body vibration exercise: influence of vibration frequency, amplitude and external load. *International Journal of Sports Medicine* 23:428–432.

Rittweger J, Mutschelknauss M, Felsenberg D (2003) Acute changes in neuromuscular excitability after exhaustive whole body vibration exercise as compared to exhaustion by squatting exercise. *Clinical Physiology and Functional Imaging* 23(2):81–86.

Roelants M, Delecluse C, Verschueren SM (2004a) Whole-body-vibration training increases knee-extension strength and speed of movement in older women. *Journal of the American Geriatric Society* 52:901–908.

Roelants M, Delecluse C, Goris M et al (2004b) Effects of 24 weeks of whole body vibration training on body composition and muscle strength in untrained females. *International Journal of Sports Medicine* 25:1–5.

Rubin C, Xu G, Judex S (2001) The anabolic activity of bone tissue suppressed by disuse is normalized by brief exposure to extremely low-magnitude mechanical stimuli. *FASEB Journal* 15:2225–2229.

Rubin C, Pope M, Fritton C et al (2003) Transmissibility of 15-Hertz to 35-Hertz vibration to the human hip and lumbar spine: Determining the physiologic feasibility of delivering low-level anabolic mechanical stimuli to skeletal regions at greatest risk of fracture because of osteoporosis. *Spine* 23:2621–2627.

Rubin C, Recker R, Cullen D et al (2004) Prevention of postmenopausal bone loss by a low-magnitude high-frequency mechanical stimuli: a clinical trial assessing compliance efficacy and safety. *Journal of Bone and Mineral Research* 19(3):343–351.

Rubin C, Capilla E, Luu YK et al (2007) Adipogenesis is inhibited by brief, daily exposure to high-frequency extremely low-magnitude mechanical signals. *Proceedings of the National Academy of Sciences of the United States of America* 104(45):17879–17884.

Runge M, Rehfeld G, Resnicek E (2000) Balance training and exercise in geriatric patients. *Journal of Musculoskeletal and Neuronal Interactions* 1(1):54–58.

Sands WA, McNeal JR, Stone MH et al (2006) Flexibility enhancement with vibration: acute and long-term. *Medicine and Science in Sports and Exercise* 38:720–725.

Sapsford R, Kelly S (2005) Pelvic floor dysfunction in low back and sacroiliac dysfunction. *In Grieve's Modern Manual Therapy*, Ch 35, pp. 507-516, Churchill Livingstone.

Schuhfried O, Mittermaier C, Jovanovic T et al (2005) Effects of whole-body vibration in patients with multiple sclerosis: a pilot study. *Clinical Rehabilitation* 19:834–842.

Skovron ML (1992) Epidemiology of low back pain. *Baillière's Clinical Rheumatology* 6:559–573.

Stewart JM, Karman C, Montgomery LD et al (2004) Plantar vibration improves leg fluid flow in perimenopausal women. *American Journal of Physiology: Integrative and Comparative Physiology* 288:623–629.

Torvinen S, Kannus P, Sievänen H et al (2002a) Effect of a vibration exposure on muscular performance and body balance. Randomized cross-over study. *Clinical Physiology and Functional Imaging* 22: 145–152.

Torvinen S, Kannu P, Sievänen H et al (2002b) Effect of four-month vertical whole body vibration on performance and balance. *Medicine and Science in Sports and Exercise* 34(9):1523–1528.

Van den Tillaar R (2006) Will whole-body vibration training help increase the range of motion of the hamstrings? *Journal of Strength Conditioning Research* 20(1):192–196.

van Nes IJ, Geurts AC, Hendricks HT et al (2004) Short term effects of whole-body vibration on postural control in unilateral chronic stroke patients: preliminary evidence. *American Journal of Physical Medicine and Rehabilitation* 83:876–884.

Vella CA (2005) Whole body vibration training. *IDEA Fitness Journal* 2(1).

Verschueren SMP, Roelants M, Delecluse C et al (2004) Effect of 6-month whole body vibration training on hip density muscle strength and postural control in postmenopausal women: a randomized controlled pilot study. *Journal of Bone and Mineral Research* 19:352–359.

Von der Heide S, Emons G, Hilgers R et al (2004) *Effect on Muscles of Mechanical Vibrations Produced by the Galileo 2000 in Combination with Physical Therapy in Treating Female Stress Urinary Incontinence.* Department Gynecology and Obstetrics, George-August-University, Gottingen, Germany.

Wakeling JM, Nigg BM, Rozitis AI (2002) Muscle activity damps the soft tissue resonance that occurs in response to pulsed and continuous vibration. *Journal of Applied Physiology* 93:1093–1103.

Ware JE, Kosinski M, Keller SD (1994) *SF-36 Physical and Mental Health Summary Scales: A User's Manual.* Health Assessment Lab, Boston, MA.

Xie L, Jacobson JM, Choi ES et al (2006) Low-level mechanical vibrations can influence bone resorption and bone formation in the growing skeleton. *Bone* 39:1059–1066.

Whole body vibration
Treatment with patients or athletes

Ingo Rembitzki

Preparation for therapy

The aim of this chapter is to offer a clinical approach to whole body vibration (WBV) and its related treatment and training possibilities in athletes as well as in patients with different diagnostic and age categories.

The proposed exercises are based on theoretical evidence from Chapters 2 and 3, as well as the clinical evidence documented in Chapter 4. In fact, one of the most important aspects of WBV is the variability in the prescription of dosage as well as the variability in the protocol used during WBV training. Moreover, this variability gives clinicians the possibility of modifying their procedure according to the type of population and the clinical outcomes attained. Most significantly, the initial assessment and subsequent reassessment define the clinical reasoning process. It appears that some groups of people and even certain subpopulations of the same condition receive more benefit from WBV than others. Therefore, it is important to match the correct dosage and protocol for each individual case based on its own clinical history.

In Chapter 4 different investigators identified parameters, variables of safety, progression and evaluation techniques which can be used not only to determine the efficacy of the treatment and training but also to highlight the clinical assessment tools which can be used to determine the selection of dosage depending upon the stage at which the patient or the athlete finds themselves. In this manner, clinical outcome not only defines a suitable population but also determines the progression of treatment or training. The spectrum of dosage will be illustrated here.

This chapter is an example of practice-based evidence derived from several years of unpublished experience. Although the following devices show a rotational device, the application of dosage applies to other types of devices as well. Importantly, evidence-based medicine has been employed by using similar exercises, protocols and guidelines to those that were discussed in Chapter 4. Since the acute and long-term effects of WBV have been extensively illustrated in Chapter 4, we will not mention them again. Interested readers should view this chapter's Appendix for a table highlighting the protocols used, outcomes attained and populations investigated in published research. Additionally, examples of assessment and reassessment tools can also be found in the Appendix. Clinical reasoning and clinical trials are a two-way street whereby each has an influence on the other, thereby defining directions for future clinical research.

Fundamental principles

The commencement of therapy takes place in the fundamental starting position. In this position the client learns to experience the feel of vibration as well as understand how to focus its effect.

Fundamental starting position (FSP)
- Feet parallel on the exercise platform.
- Bilaterally symmetrical.
- One foot-width apart with even sole contact.
- Tips of feet are rotated slightly outwards (approx 7°) similar to walking.
- Knees and hips are bent lightly.

Guidelines
- Non-slip socks or shoes;
- Use shoes with thin hard soles, which should be evaluated by the client and therapist.
- No sports shoes with cushioned or soft soles, as these absorb the vibration.
- **It is especially important to watch out for blisters in people with diabetes and/or sensory disturbances.**

Choice of frequency
- Always commence with low frequencies (5–12 Hz) and a small base of support = commence with small force.
- When familiarized and accustomed to lower frequencies continue higher frequencies (18–40 Hz) and subsequently gradually increase the amplitude.

Patient guidance

- Give hand support only when necessary.
- Observe and give verbal instructions as well as use slight contact with the client.
- Have breaks depending upon individual reactions.
- Progress training over days and weeks with gradual increases in duration and force.

Observe the reaction of the patient

- Skin colour.
- Pulse.
- Possibly blood pressure.
- Sudden movements and postural changes.

Client report/feedback

- Register verbal and spontaneous reactions.
- Do not use leading questions.
- Only after generalized questioning ('How was it?') should you ask more specific questions (e.g. pain).
- Dizziness, visual disturbances.

Guiding the patient through WBV therapy

The clients are slowly guided through the vibration treatment. Commence the initial treatment with small amplitude, lightly bent knees, slightly bending the torso and using low frequencies, e.g. 5–12 Hz. Frequency, amplitude and difficulty grading should be progressed slowly over several therapy training sessions, i.e. several exercise days and weeks.

Warm-up exercises are recommended at the start of every training therapy session

- Stimulation frequency: initially 5–12 Hz, later increased to 18–40 Hz.
- Feet positioning: parallel, e.g. at low amplitude.
- Body positioning: the knees and hips are bent gently in relaxed standing.
- Training duration: e.g. 1 min low frequency, then 1 min high frequency, 3 min back to low frequency.

Goals

- Adaptation to the vibration treatment.
- Remove any initial doubts and fears:
    - determine individual reactions, i.e. side-effects;

○ learn how the vibration can be guided into various body parts.
○ learn to control balance on the apparatus and gain confidence.
○ improve body proprioception.
○ increase circulation.

Aims for the client

- Recognize own reactions.
- Practice control over body posture.
- Feel how the trunk and joint positioning determines the spread of vibrations into different parts of the body.
- Learn how to guide the vibrations into the desired body part.

Observational objectives for the therapist

- How does the client react to manual and verbal feedback?
- Can the client steer the vibration into the different body parts?
- Are the vibrations almost symmetrical?
- Is the client able to maintain the head in a relative vibration-free state?
- Can the client maintain balance?

Safety check during treatment

- Any unusual changes in skin colour, pulse, breathing or posture?
- If necessary, measure the pulse and blood pressure.
- Does the client mention pain, dizziness, blurred vision or any other ill effects?
- Does the client react with sudden uncontrollable movements?

Preparation before the commencement of exercise

- Short explanation of the three-main variables to the client.
- Foot placement.
- Body posture (ankle, knee, hip and trunk).
- Apparatus frequency.

Instructions to the client

- Ask the client to report any unusual events.
- Inform the client that WBV can stimulate the bladder and that they should empty the bladder prior to training.
- Mention that with prolonged exercise itching can occur. This is a desirable and expected sign of increased circulation and an effect on soft tissue hormones.

- Specifically question the list of contraindications and document the checklist of clarifications.

Example of an assessment form used in the preparation for training/therapy

- Assessment form

Table 5.1 Assessment form

Surname, first name	Street name, number
Post code	Town
Telephone	
Sex	Date of birth
Age	Height

- Information on general health

Table 5.2a Information on general health

	Yes		Yes
Pacemaker	☐	Prosthesis	☐
Osteoporosis	☐	Migraine, headaches	☐
Dizziness	☐	Joint disease	☐
Muscle dysfunction	☐	Blood vessel disease, artherosclerosis	☐
Heart: cardiovascular disease	☐	Injuries or operations	☐
Neurological disturbances	☐	Pregnancy	☐

Table 5.2b

Are there any other general health issues?

- General questions

Table 5.3 General questions

What are your reasons for carrying out the training system?

- What physical activities do you undertake?

Table 5.4 What physical activities do you undertake?

Occupation
Leisure time
Sport (× per week)
Are there any other things which we should note?
Contraindications Yes ☐ No ☐ Candidate for training? Yes ☐ No ☐
Place, Date, Signature

Possible side-effects

- Blisters in the soles of the feet or on the hands, in the case of the four-point kneeling position.
- Headache.
- Itchiness in the area of stimulation.
- Nausea and dizziness.
- Short-term drop in blood pressure.
- Hypoglycaemia in people with diabetes.

The side-effects of nausea, dizziness, dropping blood pressure and excessive itchiness should not normally occur and are a sign that the training intensity is too high. Therefore, the training duration, frequency and force should be increased progressively.

Vibration training/therapy can reduce blood glucose levels and hence the training regimen should be adjusted appropriately.

Conclusion

The suggested exercises adhere to a rigid plan with specific therapeutic aims. These specifications are not intended to be too rigid but are merely suggestions which must be adapted to the individual client and to the desired therapy outcome. Here, the actual status, the individual pathology, the ability to learn and the previous experience of the client play a part. Even in patients with previous WBV experience the current status needs to be considered daily.

The posture is often described in the literature where only the knee joints are mentioned. Obviously, their position cannot be changed in isolation as the relevant positions of the hip and ankle joint determine the body posture. The upright positioning of the torso can be measured from the distance between the sternum and the pelvis. Even here, the values given are desirable aims which can be achieved over the duration of treatment. In the relaxed state, the tips of the feet are similar to during walking, i.e. turned outwards at approximately 7°. Variation in the position of the feet changes the client's distribution of the vibrations in their body and thereby affects their different muscle groups.

Vibration therapy machines are also a diagnostic aid. The stimulation of the movement platform is detected by the distribution of the vibrations. Initially, only the localized areas of the body should be activated. In order to see and feel the distribution of the vibrations on different parts of the body. The client must be touched during the treatment. Vibrations must be felt. In particular, site-specific variations should be easily detected.

The effects of muscle strength and muscle power as well as stretching and movement are located in different areas, depending on the stimulated muscle groups. Generally, circulation and body awareness will be improved by vibrations.

Guidelines and indications using examples of exercises for specific clinical conditions

The following guidelines were accumulated over several years of clinical experience.

Standard guidelines

What follows is a description of the therapeutic basis for the application of WBV for

- new therapists;
- new patients;
- the maintenance of the therapeutic treatment management plan even with a change in therapist;
- the most frequent therapeutic goals; and
- the goal-specific variation of the starting position.

The vibration therapy is suitable for:

- increasing muscle power;
- increasing muscle strength;
- improving balance and stability;

- improving movement and flexibility;
- treating osteoporosis;
- treating sarcopenia
- reducing muscle spasms and influencing muscle tone;
- treating incontinence; and
- improving blood flow.

Explanation and introduction of WBV training and WBV therapy sessions

Familiarization with the training device can be achieved in approximately 1 min with slow (5–12 Hz), subjectively comfortable frequency and middle amplitude of 'swing' (where the subjective feeling of comfort is individual and varies significantly).

S-series (S = stretching)

- Aim: Stretching to improve elasticity and joint range of motion. Stretching should be incorporated into the commencement of each training session so as to optimize the muscle elasticity.
- Vary the knee position between extended and slightly bent positions. Vibration should be felt in the body part where it is needed.
- Frequency: 10–18 Hz, subjectively comfortable 'swing frequency' (varies with the individual's posture and hence resonance frequency).
- Time/duration: Slowly attain the end position until a significant stretching can be felt; maintain this position for 10–30 s and then return to the starting position. Two or three repetitions. Repeat each exercise for 1–2 min.

B-series (B = balance)

- Aim: Improved stability, in particular for lateral balance in the ankles.
- Frequency: 5–12 Hz–the lower the frequency, the harder the exercise (varies with the individual client and posture).
- Time: Every exercise should be undertaken for 1–2 min, several repetitions of each exercise are possible, several times per day.

F-series (F = force)

- Aim: Improved muscle strength and muscle mass.
- Training progression involves increased strength and muscle mass through the addition of weights of up to 50% of body weight.

- Increase weights when more than 12 repetitions can be reached in a given time or else vary the base of support (fatigue of muscles must be reached).
- Frequency: from 25 to 40 Hz (varies with the training device).
- Time/duration: To the point of fatigue of the musculature.
- The number of sets and repetitions of these exercises should be based on what is standard practice in weight training. A 48 hour rest between training sessions is recommended.

P-series (P = power (watt) = force × velocity)

- Aim: Increase muscle power of the proximal musculature and spinal musculature.
- High frequency: 18–27 Hz.
- Duration: two or three times for 2 min, with 1-min break using walking.
- Large amplitude.
- Deep squats to 90°. The heels should remain on the vibration platform:
  - wide stance with large amplitude;
  - small up and down movement as deep as possible.
- Where insecurity exists the client can hold on; otherwise, the aim is not to hang on.

Guidelines for vibration therapy in low back pain

Therapy aims/objectives/goals

- Improved paravertebral muscle elasticity, and hence improved range of motion of the trunk.
- Synchronization of muscle function, reduction of muscle spasms, unloading of the injured structures through increased muscle strength and muscle power.

Treatment sequence

- Through the examination by the doctor and/or therapist, the aims and objectives of therapy are determined based on the deficits which need to be rectified.
- If deficits are found in strength and/or power then treatment will be directed at the P- and F-series.
- If the deficits are more to do with stability then exercises from the B-series are selected.
- Where the deficit is in the range of movement then exercises from the S-series are selected.

Examples of exercises

- The exercises should be carried out over a period of time and in all circumstances should be pain-free!
- Strength training should be adapted to the increasing strength of the client.
- The exercises should always be executed in a manner which protects the back.
- Duration of training should be of the order of 10 min.
- Two or three training sessions per week are recommended.

Table 5.5 Example of a stretching exercise

Duration of exercise	3–10 min
Frequency	5–12 Hz
Amplitude/foot placement	Low to high
Starting position	Standing, ideally not holding on. Bend the knees slightly. Direct vibration into the various body parts. Then bend the torso forwards, backwards, sideways and into rotation. Ideally, maintain the position at the end of range for 3–5 s

Table 5.6 Force and power training

Duration of each application of exercise	3–5 min
Frequency	15–30 Hz
Amplitude/foot placement	Low to middle depending upon comfort
Starting position	Exercises out of F- and P-series alternately. In principle exercise examples from B-series could also be incorporated here
Number of repetitions per series without a break	1
Break between applications	1–2 min

Additional weights can be applied through pulley apparatus or a weighted vest. This increases the muscle pre-tension and hence attains a greater training effect.

Table 5.7 Post-training relaxation

Duration of exercise	1–2 min
Frequency	5–10 Hz
Amplitude/foot placement	Low
Starting position	Loose, with slightly bent knees and without holding on, move the whole body slightly. Importantly, the soles of the feet must remain completely on the vibration platform

Guidelines for the treatment of osteoporosis/osteopenia

Treatment aims

- The aim of treatment is the improvement of muscle strength and power. Through the application of maximal muscle strength, the bones react through Wolff's law by building more bone.
- Additionally, the balance training can reduce the risk of falling, which thus decreases the likelihood of fractures.

Treatment guidelines

- Aim: The treatment of osteoporosis with WBV is a combination of the previously described S-, B-, F- and P-series.
- The treatment objectives are established from the examination by the therapist or doctor.
- If deficits in power or strength are found then exercises predominantly in the P- and F-series are selected.
- If the impairment is more in the area of coordination, then exercises are prescribed from the B-series.
- Where muscle stiffness and lack of elasticity are present, then exercises in the S-series are selected.

Exercise examples

- The exercises should be conducted over a longer period (at least 6 months) and should not in any circumstances be conducted if the person is experiencing pain.
- Strength training should be individually selected based on the concepts of progressive training.
- The exercises can be undertaken by older clients.
- Duration of a training session should be 15–20 min.
- Within 6 months, two or three training sessions per week should be undertaken, with at least 1 rest day for recovery between training sessions.

Table 5.8 Therapeutic familiarization with WBV

Duration of exercise	1–3 min
Frequency	5–12 Hz
Amplitude/foot placement	Low
Starting position	Standing with slightly bent knees. If possible without holding on. The vibration can be directed to various body parts through changes in the centre of gravity and slowly straightening the knees. Stretching exercises out of the S- and B-series

Table 5.9 Therapeutic application of WBV

Duration per application	3–5 min
Frequency	15–30 Hz
Amplitude/foot placement	Middle to high depending upon comfort
Starting position	Exercises varying between the F- and P-series. Also some of the exercises from the B-series may be appropriate
Number of applications per series without a break	1 or 2
Breaks between the applications	1–2 min

Additionally, weights on a pulley system or a weighted vest can be used. This increases the muscle pre-tension and thereby achieves a higher training effect/load.

Table 5.10 Cool down

Duration	1–2 mins
Frequency	5–10 Hz
Amplitude/foot placement	Low
Starting position	Relaxed, moving the body gently forwards and backwards with slightly bent knees while not holding on. The soles of the feet must stay fully on the vibration plate

Training with vibration for osteoporosis and osteopenia is safe. The training duration is short without any major loading of the cardiovascular system. Muscle strength and power can be built up progressively, thereby stimulating bone growth through improved muscle strength.

Guidelines for reducing the likelihood of falling

Aims of therapy

Improve the elasticity of muscles, ligaments and tendons. Thereby improvements in muscle energy absorption and storage can be achieved, which in turn improves the biomechanical and physiological parameters for muscle strength and power. The consequences of improved coordination and power are a reduction in the likelihood of falling and thereby a reduced risk of falls-related fractures.

Table 5.11	
Increased strength through	Hypertrophy of muscles and power
Reduced falls through	Improved coordination and power
Improved flexibility through	Stretching exercises which improve energy absorption and therefore muscle range of movement and hence power

Therapy methods
- Aim: Prophylaxis against falling through exercises from series P, F, B and S.
- Emphasis of therapy is determined as a result of the findings from the examination carried out by the therapist or medical doctor.
- If deficits are found in muscle power and strength then exercises are chosen from series P and F.
- If the impairment is one of coordination then the emphasis of therapy is series B.
- Where muscle stiffness and lack of elasticity are problematic then exercises from series S are given a higher priority.

Examples of exercises
The duration of treatment in clients who are at risk of falling varies between individuals.

In order to maintain/sustain mobility and power the training in these individuals should become daily routine. Progression occurs with increasing strength of the client. Divide training into sets and repetitions. At least

48 hours rest between exercise sessions are required. Balance training can be carried out several times per day. These exercises can be carried out with older individuals.

Table 5.12 Stretching/balance exercises

Duration of exercises	2–6 min
Frequency	5–12 Hz
Amplitude/foot placement	Low to middle
Starting position	In standing, carry out exercises from series B and S. The number of repetitions is individually tailored. Importantly, the whole body is gradually brought to an end-of-range position of stretching
Balance	Placing one foot alternately on the lowest position, slightly lift the other foot and hold at 5 Hz without support for 5–30 s

Table 5.13 Strength training

Duration per session	3–5 min
Frequency	25–30 Hz
Amplitude/foot placement	Middle to high depending upon comfort
Starting position	Exercises alternating from series F and P. Additionally exercises from series B can be applied
Number of repetitions	Sets of 10
Sets	3 sets per exercise
Interval between sets	10–20 s
Interval between sets	1–3 min
Additional weights	70% of individual maximal strength (the maximal strength is the weight that a person can lift once)

Additionally, weights on a pulley system or a weighted vest can be used. This increases the muscle pre-tension and thereby achieves a higher training effect/load.

Power training

Power training is attained through all series since power = force × velocity, which is a combination of coordination, balance and strength.

Table 5.14	
Starting position	Selected individually
Frequency	18–30 Hz
Amplitude	Middle to high
Duration	5–6 min
Number of repetitions	Carry out these exercises without weights, concentrating on speed and changes in direction.

Muscle power is essential to prevent falls. A reaction within milliseconds can reduce the risk of falling. The Chair Raising Test (GUG) is an appropriate parameter for measuring muscle power and therefore is convenient to assess the risk of falling.

Guidelines for impaired circulation

Treatment goals/aims/objectives

- Blood flow in the lower extremity.
- Expectations of itchiness and pins and needles in the area of training, as well as frequent redness of the skin and dilation of the veins.
- Duration of a training session: 3; maximal 9 min.
- Daily sessions are recommended.

Table 5.15a Exercise example	
Duration	3–9 min
Frequency	18–30 Hz
Amplitude/foot placement	Middle to high
Starting position	Standing, knees slightly bent. The centre of gravity of the body is slightly moved continuously and slowly

Table 5.15b

Duration of each exercise	3–5 min
Frequency	18–30 Hz
Amplitude/foot placement	Low to middle/the feet should still be maintained on the force platform even at high frequencies
Starting position	Sitting, knees bent maximally to 90°, feet hip-width apart (potentially increasing the foot pressure through pressure from the arms on the knees). Small movements through the ankles moving from tiptoes to heel positions

Guidelines for incontinence

Exercise examples

Table 5.16 Improved strength and power of the pelvic floor muscles

Strength training of the pelvic floor muscles	Muscle hypertrophy and increase sphincter control
Functional improvement	Proprioception of the pelvic floor, high repetitions
Increased flexibility through	Stretching of the abdominal muscles and pelvic floor muscles, thereby creating better storage of energy and hence muscle power and improved function

Additionally, electrotherapy, medication, weight reduction and general principles of incontinence physiotherapy should be used.

- These exercises should be conducted over a period of at least 28 weeks.
- These exercises should be carried out actively on the vibration platform.
- General exercise for pelvic floor musculature from incontinence physiotherapy should be incorporated into the treatment.
- Total duration: 20–30 min
- two or three times per week.
- For anxiety-free training, a nappy/diaper can be used.

- Signs of urine loss are an indication that the bladder is being stimulated. Initially, training should be carried out with an empty bladder and later, with increasing strength, a full bladder.

Table 5.17 Proprioceptive training for the pelvic floor

Duration	2–3 min
Frequency	10–15 Hz depending upon resonance
Amplitude/foot placement	Low, training sessions varying it with wide base of support and various fullness of bladder
Starting position	• Standing, with slightly bent knees. If possible without holding on. Through changes in the centre of gravity and slowly extending the knees, the vibration can be directed into various body parts. • Deep squats with heels on the vibration platform. • With extended knees, tighten the buttocks and stomach and then let go again.

The aim for the client is to improve proprioception of vibration in the lower abdominal muscles.

Furthermore, the pressure on the pelvic floor and bladder can be increased through breathing techniques and additional weights.

Pelvic floor training

- The positioning for pelvic floor exercises is always individual.
- Body positioning, frequency and leg positioning can optimally influence the pelvic floor.
- If no significant resonance occurs at 12 Hz then various other leg positions, starting positions and frequencies need to be assessed.
- Possible variations are shown in Table 5.18.

Table 5.18

Knee flexion/extension
Foot-width apart/amplitude
Frequency variation
Muscle pre-tension of the buttocks, pelvic floor, abdominals and legs

Exercise example

Table 5.19

Starting position	Individually optimized conscious tensioning and relaxing of the pelvic floor. Then increasing the pressure through breathing out against a closed mouth or pressure with the hands on the low abdominal region. Additionally, buttock and abdominal muscles can be activated.
Frequency	Individual 10–27 Hz
Amplitude/foot placement	Low to high
Duration	2–3 min with at least 10 repetitions of each exercise

Ability to get out of a deep squat or the ability to do activities of daily living such as lifting a heavy box can be trained.

Guidelines for the tilt table system

The tilt table allows the possibility of training at various angles between horizontal and vertical, which allows the safe and progressive loading from partial to full weight bearing.

Aim of the tilt table system

Table 5.20

Improved elasticity of the muscles, tendons and ligaments
Improved range of movement
Improved mobility
Improved muscle strength and power
Train coordination
Improve circulation
Reduce pain
Loosen spasticity and incorporate functional motor patterns
Allow a safe number of repetitions
Relearn natural movement patterns

- Acute injuries and inflammation of the tendons, ligaments and muscles requires a special treatment programme and therefore are not part of the basic protocol.
- The introduction of strength training to the human body with vibration is of the same magnitude but more controllable than walking on uneven terrain.

Clients who are unable to walk should be transferred from a wheelchair by two people onto a slanting tilt table or else from a second more highly placed bed onto the tilt table. Use safety belts to secure the client.

Individual starting positions require adjustment of the underlying surface and in particular the feet may need to be placed into the foot holsters.

For client safety in the vertical positions use the belt system above the knees.

Observe circulatory signs: skin colour, pulse, breathing. For people with diabetes, the use of glucose before the commencement of training may be indicated.

Avoid any strong vibration of the head through body positioning.

Always ensure protection against blisters.

Adjustable parameters

1. Apparatus frequency from 5–Hz to approximately 30–Hz.
2. Tilt table angle.
3. Foot placement (amplitude) from 1 to 3.
4. Body positioning.
5. Starting position (supine, prone, side lying, four-point kneeling, long sitting).
6. Changes in centre of gravity.
7. Combinations of the above parameters.

Commencement of the tilt table treatment

Table 5.21 Familiarization

Duration	1–2 min
Frequency	5–15 Hz
Amplitude/foot placement	1–3
Starting position	Individual depending upon type, stage and severity of disease. Clinical prudence and continuous assessment of affect
Angle	Individual depending upon type, stage and severity of disease. Clinical prudence and continuous assessment of affect

The starting position should be taken from the traditional schools of physiotherapy such as Bobath, Hanke concept from PNF, etc.

Exercise examples

Active stretching of muscles, tendons and ligaments is a prerequesite for successful training.

Table 5.22 Balance, coordination and motor control

Duration	15–25 min in 5-min sets, with 1-min intervals between sets. Change the starting position
Frequency	6–10 Hz
Amplitude/foot placement	1–3
Starting position	Individual
Angle	Individual
Motor control	Low frequency over a longer period. The individual movement patterns should follow a neurological training programme
Recommended training duration	6 months, three times per week

Table 5.23 Partial loading, coordination, muscle stability

Duration	Total 5–15 min
Sets	1–3 at ½–2 min
Sessions weekly	2 or 3 times
Frequency	High frequency 22–30 Hz
Amplitude/foot placement	1
Starting position	Individual
Angle	Depending upon the loading tolerance. The medically recommended partial weight bearing can be measured using scales. In this manner the appropriate angle can be chosen

Release of spasticity

The release of spasticity is individually variable from 10 to 30 Hz. Some investigations even recommend just 5 Hz.

The starting position is very important as clients should be comfortable and pain free. In some cases, the medical practitioner may include appropriate medication to reduce spasticity just prior to training.

Guidelines for weighted dumbbell training

Vibration dumbbell systems are less commonly used than the vibration platform. Vibration dumbbells can be adjusted from 5 to 40 Hz with amplitude of approximately 2.0 mm.

From the reflex-provoked muscle contraction arises an increase in strength and power, depending upon the training parameters. Improved inter- and intramuscular coordination occurs due to the nature of the cyclical and fast stimulation.

The aim of the oscillatory dumbbells is improved strength of the shoulder and elbow muscles.

Gloves should be worn before every training session in order to avoid blisters!

In a sitting or standing position, grab the dumbbells with both hands with some light pre-tension. The starting position is varied depending upon pathology. If necessary, the elbow can be flexed and supported on a table.

Familiarization

Table 5.24

Duration	1–2 min
Frequency	5–15 Hz
Starting position	Individually selected
Additional weights	None
Arm movements	Grab the dumbbells completely and move the arms in various directions. Similarly, move the neck and shoulders in various directions

Table 5.25 Strength training with the dumbbells

Duration	15–30 min
Frequency	18–40 Hz
Position	Weighted pulleys can also be used. The starting position is always individually attained through the examination process. Firstly determine the sets and repetitions by determining 70% MVC
Repetitions	2–10 repetitions with an interval between repetitions of 1 min
Sets	2–5 sets with an interval between sets of 3–5 min

Example: arm/shoulder/neck

- Aim: Increase muscle power. Move the arms in all different directions and where possible go to the end of range.
- High frequency: 18–27 Hz.
- Duration: Exercise two or three times for approx 2 mins. Shake the arms between sets.
- The firmer the grip, the stronger the vibration.

Example: shoulder stiffness

- Aim: Improvement of movement, increased muscle power.
- Frequency: 5–15 Hz (varies depending upon client and body position).
- Duration: Each exercise for 1–2 min, many repetitions of individual exercises are possible, train many times per day.
- Starting position:
  - Let the arms hang while holding the dumbbells. Frequency slowly brought to 10–15 Hz. Bend the torso forwards and move the arm diagonally and loosely back and forth.
  - The starting position should have the glenohumeral joint in the most comfortable and relaxed position.

Example: frozen shoulder

- Aim: Improved range of motion, reduced pain.
- The affected arm in either standing or sitting is taken back into extension as far as possible. If this is painful then the exercise can be carried out in the prone position on a plinth.
- Adjust the frequency to 5–15 Hz. The therapist holds the dumbbells at the motor point and slowly pushes the arm into extension while the client lightly resists and then lets slowly go.
- 5–10 repetitions in sets of 3.

Example: tennis elbow/golfer's elbow

- Aim: Reduced pain and improved range of motion.
- Starting position: The client sits in front of a table and places the affected arm at approximately 40° on the table.
- Hold the dumbbells for 1–3 min with 3–5 sets at end-of-range supination and pronation.
- Adjust the frequency to 10–18 Hz.
- Afterwards the same movement for 1 min at 30 Hz.
- Break of 20 s, then with the elbow in extension 3 × 10 repetitions at 15 Hz of flexion and extension.
- Training should normalize muscle tone, reduce pain and reconstitute normal movement.
- In the case of acute inflammation of less than 6 weeks' duration, the correct application should result in resolution of symptoms.
- If the diagnosis seems to be unclear, the therapist or medical doctor should be consulted.

Exercise proposals

Basic positioning

Description

- Starting position for adapting to the vibration.
- Preparation for further exercises.

Position of feet

- Tight position of the feet: symmetrical and parallel.
- Tips of feet approx. 7° to the outside.
- One foot-width apart.
- Standing with feet flat, with force evenly distributed on the exercise platform.

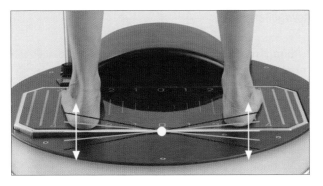

Figure 5.1

Body positioning

- Upright.
- Facing the front.
- Large leg joints slightly bent.
- Arms hanging relaxed.
- Support at the beginning only if feeling insecure.

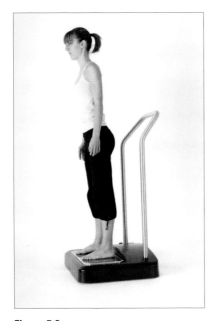

Figure 5.2

Execution, exercise duration and stimulation frequency

- Remain in the described position.
- Only small variation in the posture.
- 1 min at low frequency (5–12 Hz) subjectively acceptable frequency and symmetrical position of the feet, then 1 min at high frequency (18–40 Hz), then again 1 min at low frequency (5–12 Hz).
- Depending upon body mass and stiffness (muscle tone) frequency and amplitude can be individually tailored.

Objective

- Adjust the client to the vibration.
- Optimize the neuromuscular processes, safety through postural control enhancement.
- Improve circulation and body awareness.
- Learn how the vibrations are distributed and controlled in the body.

Comments: Recommendations before each treatment

The exercises need to be introduced as a concept of learning. The clients must learn to recognize and to specifically control the connection between minimal changes in the posture and the vibrations in the different parts of the body. Self-awareness comes from experience of voluntary control and guided movements.

Weight shift to the forefoot

Description

Starting position from the basic position moving the critical point of the body mass over the forefoot–the heels are raised at the same time.

Position of feet

- Symmetrical parallel foot positioning/small amplitude.
- Point the feet 7° outwards.
- Initially 1 foot-width apart and gradually increase this.
- Finally stand on the forefoot while raising the heels.

Body positioning

- Upright, large leg joints slightly bent.
- Arms hanging relaxed.
- Support at the beginning only if insecure.

Execution of the exercise

- Starting from the basic position move the weight by slightly bending the torso or translate movement of the torso slowly ahead onto the front feet.
- Simultaneously lift the heels alternately and to different heights.
- Raise the torso by different degrees: observe the distance between thorax and hip.

Training duration and stimulation frequency

- 1 min at low frequency (5–12 Hz), subjective acceptable frequency and tight foot position.
- Then 1 min of high frequency (18–40 Hz).
- Then 1 min of low frequency (5–12 Hz).
- The duration of the exercise is varied, depending on the patient and the entire programme.

Aim/objective/goal

- Learn how the vibrations can be controlled in different parts of the body. Foot and calf muscles are especially stimulated in the forefoot position. By decreasing the support base higher demands are directed to the control of the critical point of the mass and thereby improvements in balance are achieved.
- Reduce the possibility of a fall.

Comments/notes

The position of the forefoot and especially the dynamic change of the body's critical point the forefoot is more difficult than the basic position. Care is to be taken when leading to the final position. Teach safety. By very slowly raising the demand the client learns that the variation of the position of the feet stimulates other body regions. Move the vibrations to the lower leg.

Weight shift to the heel

Description

- From the basic position move the critical point over the heel, knees straight, lift the forefoot.

Foot placement

- Symmetrical foot placement.
- Feet pointed lightly outwards at 7°.

- Initially approximately 1 foot-width apart and then gradually increase this.
- Finally, stand on the heels, lightly lifting the forefeet.

Body positioning

- Upright, large joints of the legs nearly extended.
- Allow the arms to hold loosely.
- Only hang on if unsure/insecure/unsteady.

Execution of exercise

Starting from the basic position move the weight very slowly in the direction of the heels while simultaneously lifting the forefoot to various degrees alternately. This results in large variation in the distribution of vibration. Lift slightly. Balance on the heels is very difficult to control because the sideways rotation through pronation and supination cannot function to compensate for the perturbations in body movement. Initially, the clients often need to hold on to a support and can stand freely for only a few seconds. The therapist must give support/assistance.

Training duration and stimulation frequency

- 1 min at low frequency (5–15 Hz), subjectively acceptable frequency with a small amplitude.
- Then 1 min at higher frequency (15–30 Hz).
- Then again at lower frequency (5–15 Hz).

Aim/objective/goal

- Learn how the vibrations can be directed to different parts of the body: vibrations are preferentially directed to the paravertebral muscle structure. The support base and major elimination of the effect of supination and pronation makes this experience more difficult, which thereby makes the exercise more difficult and therefore challenges the balancing experience.
- Reduce the risk of falling.

Comments

The control of this position is much more demanding/challenging than that in the basic position or the forefoot positions. Careful guidance is needed. Impart safety through learning. Very slowly raise the demand. Possibly stand without support for only a few seconds; intermittent support is also part of this. For clients with reduced balance it is advisable to offer constant support. Clients learn by changing the critical point and the position of the feet; other parts of the body can be stimulated, thereby directing vibration into the torso, and especially into the back. While on the edge of the heel the centre of gravity is placed on the hip joints.

Squatting with/without weights

Description
- Feet spread apart–standing in a bent position.
- Stimulation of the hip–pelvis–back musculature through the use of weights, as well as shoulders and arms.

Foot placement
- Feet spread apart, medium amplitude.
- Pointing the feet 20–30° outwards.
- Feet flat with even distribution of weight on the training platform.

Body positioning
- Bent position, knees bent strongly, torso far to the front, back straight buttocks stretched back.
- Weight in both hands, with arms stretched out at different lengths.
- The stretching of the torso forwards and the pelvis back with bent hip joints must be watched closely.
- Scapula directed medially and inferiorly.

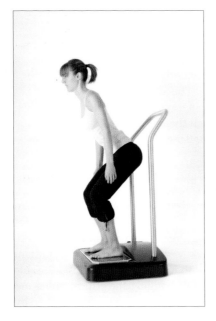

Figure 5.3

Execution

- Stay in this position, as deep as possible, gently moving up and down. Arms with weights are stretched forwards differently so as to obtain a torque (rotational moment).
- Variation: Large amplitude of going up and down, slowly 5 s down, 5 s up.

Exercise duration and stimulation frequency

- After the progressive build-up of treatment, high frequency (18–40 Hz), 1–2 min. Fatigue of the muscles must be reached.
- Potentially after a few minutes rest, the exercise may be repeated.
- Frequency of treatment: two or three times per week, depending on fitness level; daily may be possible.

Aim/objective/goal

- Improvement of muscle strength and muscle power of the hip–pelvic–back musculature.
- Improvement of the range in movement of the hip, knee and ankle.
- Stimulation of the arm and shoulder musculature.
- Stimulus for bone growth.

Comments

A reduction of strength and power in the hip musculature is, next to balance, the most important neuromuscular falls risk, which can be fateful in older people. Muscle fatigue should be reached. In the presence of knee problems the exercises should be progressed slowly.

Forward bending of the torso increases the torque of the torso in relation to the hip joint and pre-stretching of the gluteus maximus.

Torso bending/torso extending

Description

- With extended or slightly bent knees bend the torso down and forward.

Foot positioning

- Comfortable, not too narrow foot positioning with middle amplitude.
- Feet rotated approximately 7° outwards, more than 1 foot-width apart.
- Even distribution on the platform.

Body posture

- Stretch the knees as much as possible.
- Arms and legs are in relaxed hanging position.

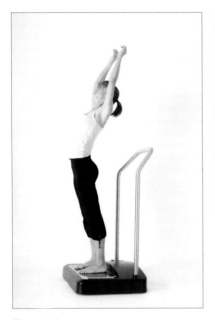 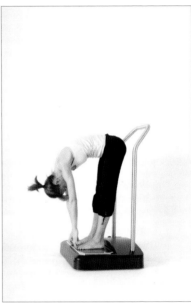

Figure 5.4   **Figure 5.5**

Execution, duration and stimulation frequency

- From a straight standing position very slowly, over 8 s, bend the torso forward, not with momentum or force. Do not simultaneously rotate. Subsequently, lift the arms over the head and with a stretched spine reach upwards.
- Fingertips to the floor, stay down for 10–30 s, and move slightly up and down, carefully feeling into the body.
- Repeat this exercise two or three times. Change the stimulation frequency in the mid-region depending upon the mass and stiffness of the client. Be guided by the range of movement and the sense of well-being.

Aim/objective/goal

- Stretching the calves, hamstrings and back extensors. With the torso stretching, the hip, this allows more room for increasing the moment arm. The greater the moment arm and the greater the force, the greater the absorption of potential energy.
- Pain relieving, muscle relaxation.

Comments

The importance of stretching has been dealt with earlier and should be explained the physiotherapist. With improved range of movement, an improved kinaesthetic awareness should follow. Improved range of movement leads to muscle relaxation, prevention of pain and eleviation/reduction of pain.

Both exercises are often discussed controversially. The correct execution of these exercises requires careful guidance and instruction by the therapist. The patient must learn to carry out these movements with finesse and good body awareness. The boundaries of balance and being pain-free must be carefully monitored.

In cases of back and intervertebral disc pathology it is wise for the therapist to discuss these exercises with the treating physician.

Pelvic tilting

Description

- Tilt the pelvis forwards and backwards with slightly bent knees.

Foot placement/positioning

- Feet hip-width apart, slightly rotated outwards, flat with even distribution of force on the training platform, at middle amplitude.

Body positioning

- Knees slightly bent, the hands hold the pelvis near the hips. The hands feel and guide the pelvic tilting manoeuvre.

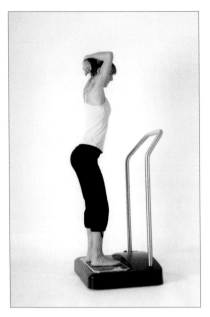

Figure 5.6

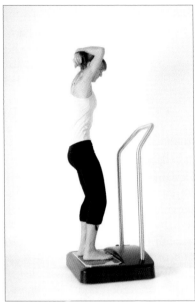

Figure 5.7

Execution, duration and stimulation frequency

- Very slowly tilt the pelvis. Maintain a constant position of the knees and attempt to isolate the movement to the pelvis.
- Duration: Approximately 1–3 min, middle stimulation frequency varying with the mass and stiffness of the client.
- Guidance dependent upon pelvic range of motion and sense of awareness.

Aim/objective/goal

- Stretching and selective movement in the region of the lumbar spine to improve torso control.
- Pain reduction, muscle relaxation.

Comments/notes

Stiffness in the hips is not only a problem among soccer players. Elasticity/pliability in the region of the hips and control of the upper body over the hips is the principal function for fluid motion of gait and body control.

Trunk side bending (A) and trunk rotation (B)

- (A) Move the hand down the side of the leg in the frontal plane; the upper body does not turn or bend.
- (B) In erect standing the trunk is turned left and right around the longitudinal axis horizontal plane.

Foot positioning

- Comfortable, not too narrow stance, small amplitude, feet turned approximately 7° outwards, more than 1 foot-width apart.
- Feet flat with even distribution of force on the vibration platform.

Body positioning

- Knee extended as much as possible.
- (A) Arms hanging left and right, hands on the trousers seam.
- (B) The arm in the direction of movement is abducted to 90°, palm down. The opposite arm is bent in front of the chest, the palm directs the shoulder to the back.

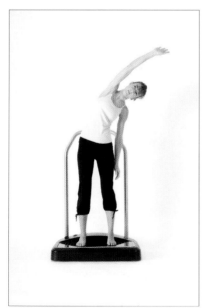 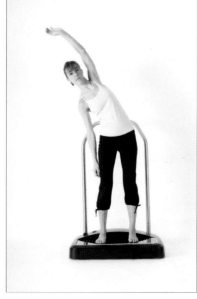

Figure 5.8 **Figure 5.9**

Execution, duration and stimulation frequency

- (A) In the erect position tilt the trunk sideways, without momentum or force, over 8 s.
- In the frontal plane, attempt to maintain pure lateral flexion, and therefore do not rotate simultaneously. Use the fingertips to bend sideways along the seams of the trousers.
- (B) Very slowly turn to the left and then the right, the head following the outstretched arm in the frontal plane, and stay at the end of range for 10–30 s, while moving very slightly up and down, feeling carefully into the end of range.

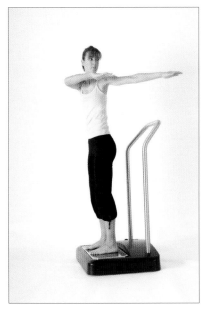 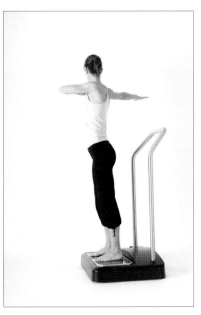

Figure 5.10   **Figure 5.11**

- Repeat two or three times.
- Stimulation frequency is dependent on the resonance.
- Be guided by range of motion and perceived comfort.

Aim/objective/goal

- (A) Stretching the side trunk and pelvic muscles.
- (B) Stretching the obliquely oriented trunk and pelvic musculature.
- By increasing the stretch, the displacement increases, which results in greater absorption of potential energy for greater

rapidity in movement and improved power. Better stretching leads to pain reduction and muscle relaxation.

Comments/notes

The importance of stretching has been explained earlier and should be taught to the client. Through improved range of motion, an improved subjective feeling of well-being should ensue. Improved range of movement leads to muscle relaxation and pain prevention as well as pain reduction.

One-leg standing

Description

- The client stands on one leg on one side of the vibration platform at various frequencies.

Foot placement/positioning

- Parallel, middle or high amplitude, foot pointing forward.
- Amplitude is progressively increased.

Body positioning

- Upright, bending lightly the joints of the stance leg.
- Free leg held up in a relaxed manner.
- Arms balanced for support.

Execution, duration and stimulation frequency

- Maintain the position and try to move gently up and down.
- 1 min at low frequency (5–12 Hz), perceived pleasant frequency, then 1 min at high frequency (18–40 Hz), then 1 min at low frequency (5–12 Hz).
- The distance to the mid-axis can be varied.

Aim/objective/goal

- Improve the balance, especially to the side.
- Reduce the risk of falling.

Comments/notes

As bipeds we spend 80% of our time on one leg: the critical aspect of walking is the control of the lateral gravitational forces. This is exactly what is being practised here.

When practising balance, both low- and high-frequency stimulation should be applied.

Frequency of balance training: in the selected position and frequency, which is considered difficult = that doesn't feel safe.

One-leg standing 90° on a side altering device

Description
- The client stands on one leg on the platform with the foot at 90° to the vibration axis.

Foot placement
- 90° to the axis, with the foot pointing laterally. Here, the compensatory movements are further from the axis and hence the demand on the balancing mechanisms is higher.

Body positioning
- Erect, joints of the stance leg bent slightly, the free leg held in a relaxed manner.
- Arms balanced over the possible support.

Execution, duration and stimulation frequency
- Maintain the position and move gently up and down.
- 1 min at low frequency (5–15 Hz), subjectively comfortable, then 1 min at high frequency (15–30 Hz), then another minute at low frequency (5–15 Hz).
- Vary the distance to the mid-axis.

Aim/objective/goal
- Improve the balance forwards and backwards.
- Reduce the risk of falling.

Squat with adductors or abductor tension

Description
- Wide base of support and bent position while standing.
- Stimulation of the hip musculature and the adductors by pressing a ball between the knees, the abductors by pulling them apart against the resistance of an elastic band around the knees.

Foot positioning
- Wide symmetrical stance, middle amplitude, feet turned 20–30° outwards.
- Feet flat with even distribution of force.

Body positioning

- Bent position, knees bent, trunk bent a long way forwards, buttocks stretched back.
- Engagement of elastic band or ball.

Execution

- Staying in this position, go down as deeply as possible, and move slightly up and down.
- Variation: Press a ball between the knees.
- Variation: Use an elastic band to pull knees apart.
- Fatigue of the muscles should occur within 1–2 min.

Duration and frequency

- After progressive training, high frequency (18–40 Hz), for 1–2 min, with either elastic bands or ball training with the knees.
- Potentially after a few minutes rest, the exercise can be repeated one more time.
- Training frequency per week: two or three times per week; where the client is fit, daily sessions may be possible.

Aim/objective/goal

- Maintain and increase the strength and power of the hip muscles, and the back muscles and specifically also the abductors and adductors.
- Improved balance.
- Reduced risk of falling.

Comments/notes

When we are walking or running and we are transferring the weight rapidly from one leg to the next, then the abductors of the stance leg control the torque that the trunk creates to the swing side, while the adductors through the pelvis and abdominal muscles counter pelvic torsion and trunk lateral flexion. Thereby, the abductors and adductors are the main muscles of the frontal plane.

Deep squat

Description

- Bent, wide base of support; and
- Stimulation of the hip musculature.

Feet positioning

- Wide symmetrical foot positioning, middle to large amplitude, feet rotated 20–30° outwards. Feet flat with even force distribution on the vibration platform.
- With increasing force, the distance between the legs can be increased.

Body positioning

- Squat, large leg joints heavily bent. Trunk straight and bent a long way forward, with the pelvis stretched back.
- With progressive training, try to go as deep as possible into the squat.

Execution

- Maintain the position as low as possible and try to move gently up and down.
- Variation: Slowly up and down, 3 s up and 3 s down.
- Fatigue of the musculature should be reached.
- Distance between the legs can be changed depending upon the fatigue. Training can be augmented or ameliorated.

Duration and frequency

- With progressive training higher frequencies (12–40 Hz) can be used, for 1–2 mins.
- Potentially repeat the exercises after a few minutes rest.
- Training frequency two or three times per week.

Aim/objective/goal

- Maintain and increase the strength and power of the hip, leg and back musculature. Through increasing strength, stimulation of bone growth is improved.
- Improve the range of movement of the hip, knee and ankle; hence, improved energy absorption and increased speed of movement (kinetic energy).

Comments/notes

The reduction of strength and power around the hip musculature is, after side balance, one of the most important neuromuscular factors in preventing falls. Optimal training stimulation should incorporate reaching muscle fatigue. With knee problems care should be taken with progression.

The rule for all squat positioning is as follows: by bending the trunk forwards the torque created on the gluteal muscles is high. Therefore, training these muscles is highly relevant in the sit–stand (GUG) test as part of the assessment of the risk of falling and maintenance of independence.

One-leg squat

Description
- Standing on one bent leg.
- Strong stimulation of the hip, thigh and back muscles.

Foot positioning
- The long axis of the feet should be parallel at small amplitude. With increasing strength the amplitude can be increased.

Body positioning
- Bend the knees of the stance leg as much as possible, with the trunk forwards and the pelvis back.
- Bring the centre of gravity of the trunk forwards to the axis of rotation of the hip, thereby increasing the torque around the hip.
- During progression try to go as deep as possible into the squat.
- Hold on so that the force is transferred with optimal movement coordination and optimal joint congruence, thereby reducing the risk of injury.

Execution
- Maintain the position as low as possible, and then in this position try to move lightly up and down.
- Variation: Slowly move up and down, 4 s up and 4 s down.

Duration and frequency
- After progressive training higher frequency (18–30 Hz) can be used, for 1–2 min. Potentially, after 1-min rest, the exercise can be repeated once. Then repeat on the other leg.
- Fatigue should be reached within 1–2 mins.
- Training frequency per week: two or three times per week.

Aim/objective/goal
- Maximum increase in muscle mass, muscle strength and muscle power of the hip, leg and back muscles.

- Improved range of movement of the hip, knee and ankle joints.
- Stimulation of bone growth around the hips.

Comments/notes

Bone structure is continually remodelled as a result of muscle forces. Avoidance of hip fractures can be achieved through the maximal metabolic stress of fatigue, which results in improved strength and power and muscle mass.

In the presence of knee problems care must be taken to progress slowly. Forward movement of the trunk increases the torque on the gluteal musculature. The relevance of training these muscles has been shown in the sit–stand (GUG) test for balance training.

Trunk horizontal

Description
- Wide stance with legs fairly straight, bend the trunk forward.

Foot positioning
- Middle amplitude, feet symmetrical, feet turned slightly outwards. Feet flat with even force distribution.

Body positioning
- Knees straight, hips at 90°, trunk stretched pelvis back, head placed lightly into the neck.
- The arms hang loosely or stretched forwards.

Execution
- Maintain the position. Arm position can be varied.
- Potentially hold a baton in both hands and stretch forward.

Duration and frequency
- With progression high frequency (15–30 Hz) can be used, for 1–2 min. Muscle fatigue should be reached.
- Potentially after a 1- to 2-min break the exercise can be repeated.
- Training frequency per week: two or three times per week.

Aim/objective/goal

- Maintain and increase strength and power in the gluteal and back muscles.
- Stretch the posterior leg muscles.
- Stimulate bone growth.

Comments

Through the forward positioning of the trunk a maximal torque is achieved around the hip joint which is countered by maximal gluteal activation.

Strengthening exercises

Upper limb

Triceps muscles

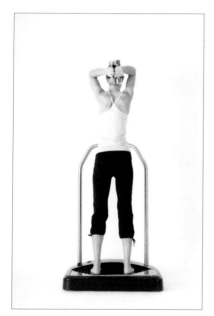 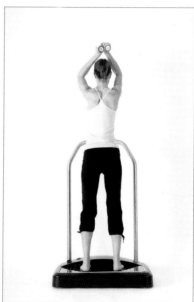

Figure 5.12 **Figure 5.13**

Biceps/triceps muscles

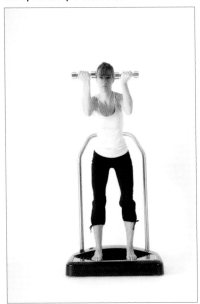 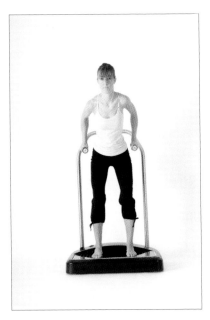

Figure 5.14   **Figure 5.15**

Whole arm muscle

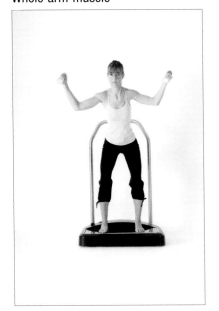

Figure 5.16

Push up

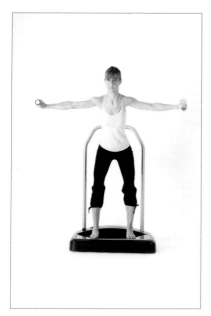

Figure 5.17

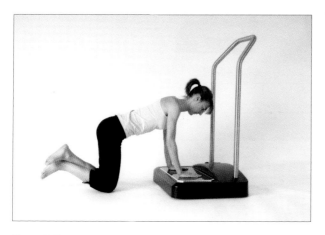

Figure 5.18

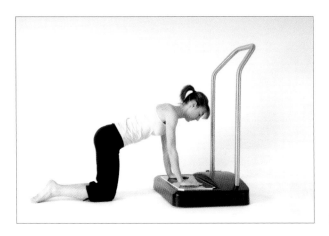

Figure 5.19

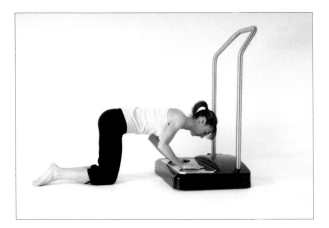

Figure 5.20

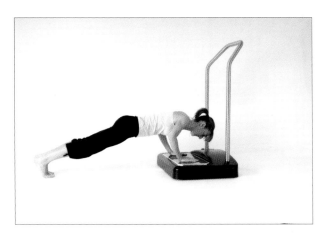

Figure 5.21

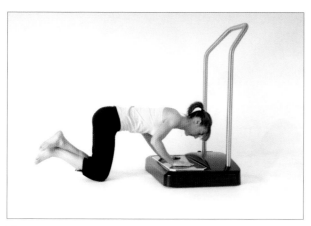

Figure 5.22

Upper body

Abdominal muscles

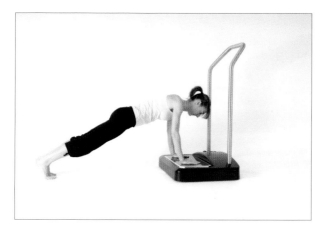

Figure 5.23

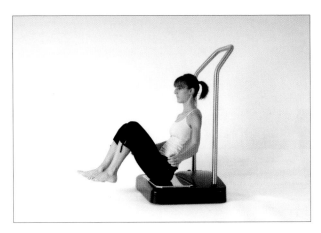

Figure 5.24

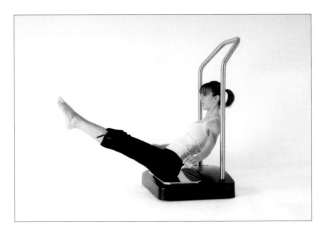

Figure 5.25

With theraband

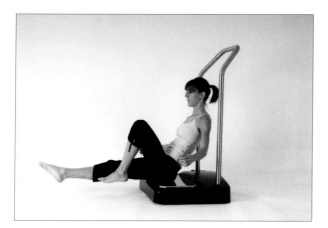

Figure 5.26

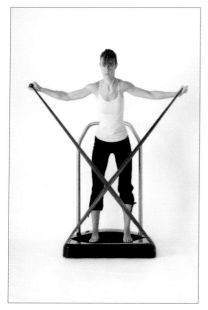

Figure 5.27

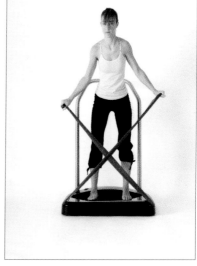

Figure 5.28

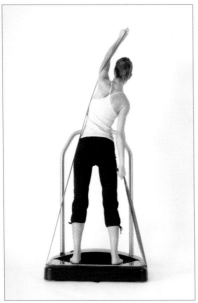
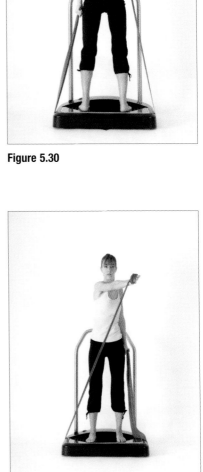

Figure 5.29

Figure 5.30

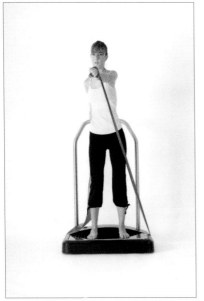

Figure 5.31

Figure 5.32

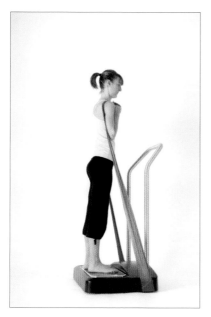

Figure 5.33

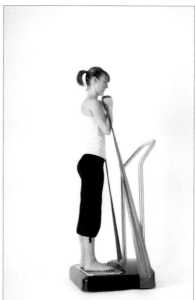

Figure 5.34

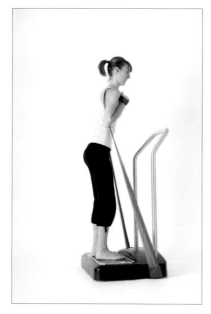

Figure 5.35

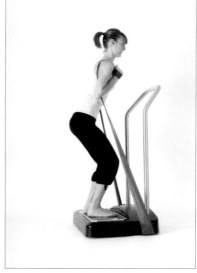

Figure 5.36

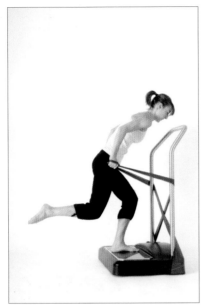

Figure 5.37

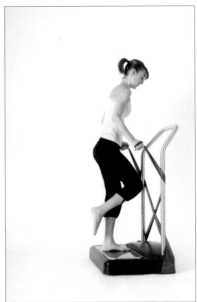

Figure 5.38

WBV as a warm-up prior to sport
Effects on flexibility

Alfio Albasini

Whole body vibration and the effect on flexibility: a review

Whole body vibration (WBV) has been advocated as a warming-up device prior to sport. It is thought that WBV has an influence on muscle length and, muscle blood flow as well as an impact on soft-tissue viscoelastic resonance.

Nazarov and Zilinsky (1984) were the first researchers to start to experiment with the effect of vibration training (VT) on flexibility. They demonstrated that vibration stretching could increase the range of motion (ROM) in the shoulder of male gymnasts. Other authors followed these interesting preliminary results.

Issurin et al (1994) tested the effect of vibratory stimulation training on maximal force and flexibility in athletes. Twenty-eight male physical education students, aged between 19 and 25 years, underwent a localized vibration training, 44 Hz and 3-mm amplitude, applied through cables during exercise for three times a week for 3 weeks. The subjects stretched during the application of vibration by placing their foot onto a ring suspended from an overhead vibrating device. The vibrating ring provided stimulation for the leg in the ring while the subject stretched the leg. Each subject placed their foot into the ring and stretched for 6–7 s, which was followed by 3–4 s of rest, and this was repeated two to four times. The subjects also performed static stretching exercises with the same parameters as the vibration stretching. The group who underwent VT had a mean increase of 8.7% in the legs split compared with a mean average of

2.4% increase in the conventional group and only 1.2% in the placebo group. An even bigger result was seen for the trunk flexion component. The flexibility group showed a mean gain of 43.6% compared with 19.2% in the conventional group and 5.8% in the placebo group. Issurin et al (1994) concluded that vibration exercise resulted not only in an increase in the maximal strength, but also in increase in flexibility, much greater than in conventional training procedures. They stated also that the gain rate in strength, seen in their research, differed from the gain rate in flexibility during vibration stimulation. Issurin et al (1994) also measured what is called the flex-and-reach test (Lycholat 1990), which measures the distance between the fingertips and a horizontal mark at foot level when subjects flex their trunk–hip joint forward. Obviously this test includes the flexibility of several joints of the trunk and therefore this may result in a larger increase in ROM when compared with other studies where only one part of the body, or one joint, is tested. The increased flexibility measured by the author ranged from 10.9 cm, before training, to 15.65 cm after VT. As an underlying mechanism, for the effect on flexibility, they proposed that the Golgi tendon organs, which are sensitive to active tension (via Ib pathways), stimulated from the vibration, would evoke an autogenic inhibition of contraction resulting in relaxation of the muscle. They postulated also that vibration of contracting muscles would prevent squeezing of the capillaries which normally occurs during muscle contraction. Hence, the rhythmical oscillation of the vibration would elicit a mechanical pump effect on the intramuscular tissue and therefore cause an increase in blood flow and enhance the local muscle temperature. They concluded by suggesting that the alleviation of pain by vibration may also be a component during the active stretching regimens which elicits such good results.

Van den Tillaar (2006) assessed whether WBV training on a vibration platform would have a positive effect on flexibility training (contract–relax method) by enhancing the ROM of the hamstring musculature, which is a muscle group where frequent muscle strains occur. Nineteen physical education students (12 women and 7 men, mean age 21.5 ± 2.0 years) were randomly allocated to either a WBV group or a control group. Both groups underwent a 4-week programme, where they were stretching, according to the contract–relax method (three times with a 5-s isometric contraction on each leg followed by 30 s of static stretching), three times per week. Before each stretching exercise the WBV group would stand on a vibration platform, Nemes Bosco system (28 Hz with 10-mm amplitude) for 30 s, six times per training session in a squat position with knees bent at 90° of flexion. The result demonstrated a significant increase in hamstring flexibility by 14% in the control group and 30% in the WBV training group.

The authors explained their results with three possible mechanisms. One possibility would be enhanced local blood flow which takes place immediately (9 min) after VT (Kerschan-Schindl et al 2001). Increased blood flow can generate additional heat which can facilitate ROM during stretching exercise because muscle elasticity is enhanced. The second mechanism may be related to the tonic vibration reflex. Vibration can cause soft-tissue deformation which is capable of activating muscle spindles (Wakeling et al 2003) and may lead to an enhancement of the stretch–reflex loop (Cardinale & Bosco 2003). The frequency used in the present study was 28 Hz, which reflects the natural frequency of the quadriceps (Wakeling et al 2003), and therefore the authors hypothesized that the stretch reflex of the quadriceps muscles was stimulated to damp the induced frequency. Cardinale and Lim (2003) demonstrated that WBV transmitted through a vibrating platform at 30 Hz, in half-squat position, was able to produce the highest electromyograph (EMG) activity in vastus lateralis of the quadriceps compared with non-vibrating conditions. Cardinale and Bosco (2003) suggested that VT appears to inhibit activation of the antagonist muscles through Ia-inhibitory neurones. Thus, activating the quadriceps muscles would relax the hamstring muscles and thereby have a positive influence on the stretching exercise. Cardinale and Lim (2003) also stated that vibrations were perturbations perceived by the central nervous systems which modulates the stiffness of the stimulated muscle groups. The reflex muscle activity could then be considered a neuromuscular tuning response to minimize soft-tissue vibrations. These responses are individual and therefore related to individual capabilities in damping external perturbations in order to avoid resonance effects. The third mechanism mentioned by Van den Tillaar (2006) is the proprioceptive feedback potentiation of inhibition of pain and increased pain threshold. As stated already by Issurin et al (1994), subjects reported that the sensation of pain was reduced within 10–15 s of beginning the static stretching during vibration.

Sands et al (2006) in their study wanted to determine whether vibration-aided static stretching could enhance ROM more than static stretching alone, in the forward split position. Ten young male gymnasts, participating in intensive gymnastics training (age = 10.1 ± 1.5 years), were randomly assigned to experimental ($n = 5$) and control ($n = 5$) groups. The test consisted of performing what is called the 'forward split position' for stretching on the vibration devices in two different positions. In the first position the athlete places their forward leg on the vibrating device such that the posterior calf area is supported by the device (Figure 6.1). In the second position the gymnast assumes a lunge position with the rear thigh directly on top of the vibrating device (Figure 6.2). The height of the anterior iliac spine of the pelvis was measured at the lowest split position.

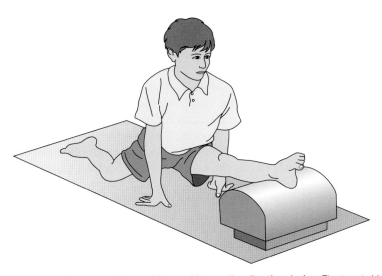

Figure 6.1 **Forward split stretching position on the vibration device.** The targeted leg in this position is the forward leg.

Reprinted from Sands WA, McNeal JR, Stone MH et al (2006) Flexibility enhancement with vibration: acute and long-term. *Medicine and Science in Sports and Exercise* 38:720–725, with permission.

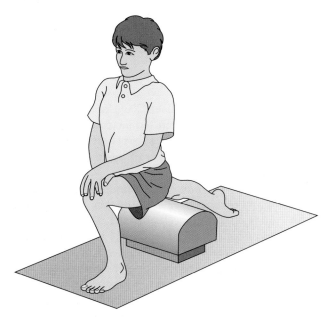

Figure 6.2 **Forward split stretching position on the vibration device.** The targeted leg in this position is the rear leg.

Reprinted from Sands WA, McNeal JR, Stone MH et al (2006) Flexibility enhancement with vibration: acute and long-term. *Medicine and Science in Sports and Exercise* 38:720–725, with permission.

The protocol consisted in stretching of the forward and rear legs to the point of discomfort for 10 s followed by 5 s of rest, repeated four times on each leg (right and left) resulting in 1 min of total stretching in each position, for a total of 4 min for one complete session of stretching. The experimental group stretched with the device turned on; the control group stretched with the device turned off. The devices were floor units which consisted of a heavy base to which was attached an upper section that was vibrated by an electric motor that resulted in a sinusoidal vibration frequency of approximately 30 Hz and an approximate displacement of 2 mm. A pre-test was followed by an acute phase post-test; thereafter, a second post-test measurement was performed following 4 weeks of treatment. The acute effect of the vibration treatment resulted in immediate and dramatic increases in forward split flexibility for both legs ($p < 0.05$). The long-term effects showed that one split side reached a statistically significant increase in ROM only on the right rear leg ($p < 0.05$), whereas the other did not. Sands et al (2006) stated in their analysis that the lack of statistical significance on one side during the long-term post-test may have been the result of the increased variability of the splits observed in the control group. The present study is similar to that of Issurin et al (1994) regarding the period of time and the protocol of stretching used. Sands et al (2006) concluded the study, mentioning that vibration effects on range of motion enhancement are incompletely understood and may provide a window into further understanding of the role of muscle spindles, Golgi tendon organs and the importance of higher central nervous system influence on polysynaptic reflexes, and other aspects of motor control.

Kinser et al (2008) wanted to test the effects of simultaneous vibration stretching on flexibility and explosive strength in competitive female gymnasts. Twenty-two female athletes (age = 11.3 ± 2.6 years) composed the experimental vibration stretching (VS) group, which performed two tests: flexibility and jumping. There were four control groups whose constituents were subpopulations of the VS group who did stretching only (SF) ($n = 7$) and vibration only (VF) ($n = 8$). Explosive strength-control groups were stretching only (SES) ($n = 8$) and vibration only (VES) ($n = 7$). The vibration device [similar to that used by Sands et al (2006)], 30 Hz, 2-mm displacement, was applied to four sites, four times for 10 s, with 5 s of rest in between as in based on the same protocol [Sands et al (2006)]. Right and left forward split (RFS and LFS) flexibility was measured by the distance between the ground and the anterior superior iliac spine. A force plate (sampling rate, 1000 Hz) recorded countermovement and static jump characteristics. Explosive strength variables included flight time, jump height, peak force, instantaneous forces and rates of force development. The results demonstrated a statistically significant increased flexibility (p)

with large effect sizes (d) in both the right forward split (p =1.28, d = 0.67) and left forward split (p = 2.35, d = 0.72) (Figure 6.3, Table 6.1). A very interesting finding in this research is that the addition of vibration to stretching not only increases flexibility but also maintains explosive strength (e.g., jumping ability). This observation is important considering that the athletes were already warmed up, as evidenced by the lack of change in ROM among the groups not receiving any vibration. As a possible mechanism affecting flexibility by vibration and stretching, the author mentioned decreased musculotendinous stiffness, muscular antagonist inhibition and increased pain threshold. It is important to note that, in the present study, stretching alone resulted in a loss of jump performance; however, the addition of acute vibration seems to have preserved the ability to express explosive strength (Tables 6.1 and 6.2).

This has already been seen in previous studies in which stretching resulted in decreased explosive strength in force production and rate of force development. Similar findings were described by Cardinale and Lim (2003). In their study, vibration combined with stretching did not increase the jumping performance. Moreover it caused no loss of explosive strength, which means that vibration and stretching are enhancing flexibility while not impairing explosive strength. The authors concluded the paper advo-

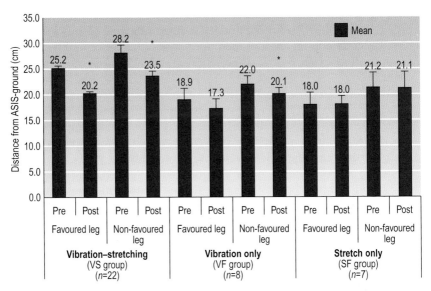

Figure 6.3 Changes in flexibility in relation to the athlete's favoured leg, dictated by the rearward leg in the split position. Statistically different means before vs after, Bonferroni adjusted p value.

Reprinted from Kinser AM, Ramsey MW, O'Bryant HS et al (2008) Vibration and stretching effects on flexibility and explosive strength in young gymnasts. *Medicine and Science in Sports and Exercise* 40(1):133–140.

Table 6.1 Flexibility results

Group	Test	Trial	Mean height (cm)	Effect size (d)	t-test (p)
VS (N = 22)	Right forward split	Pre vibration–stretching	26.2 ± 7.1		
VS (N = 22)		Post vibration–stretching	21.4 ± 7.0*	0.67	$1.28 \times 10^{-7*}$
VS (N = 22)	Left forward split	Pre vibration–stretching	27.5 ± 7.1		
VS (N = 22)		Post vibration–stretching	22.6 ± 6.8*	0.72	$2.35 \times 10^{-7*}$
SF (N = 7)	Right forward split	Pre stretch, no vibration	19.4 ± 5.0		
SF (N = 7)		Post stretch, no vibration	19.0 ± 4.9	0.08	2.49×10^{-1}
SF (N = 7)	Left forward split	Pre stretch, no vibration	20.3 ± 5.4		
SF (N = 7)		Post stretch, no vibration	20.6 ± 5.6	0.05	6.37×10^{-1}
VF (N = 8)	Right forward split	Pre vibration, no stretch	20.2 ± 6.8		
VF (N = 8)		Post vibration, no stretch	18.5 ± 6.7*	0.25	$6.98 \times 10^{-3*}$
VF (N = 8)	Left forward split	Pre vibration, no stretch	20.8 ± 5.9		
VF (N = 8)		Post vibration, no stretch	18.9 ± 6.7	0.30	$2.6 \times 10^{-2*}$

*Statistically different before vs after treatment (Bonferroni adjusted *P* value). Table (mean ± SD) represents results of the flexibility tests from all groups: vibration–stretching (VS), stretching only (SF), and vibration only (VF).
Reprinted from Kinser AM, Ramsey MW, O'Bryant HS et al (2008) Vibration and stretching effects on flexibility and explosive strength in young gymnasts. *Medicine and Science in Sports and Exercise* 40(1):133–140, with permission from

Table 6.2 Static jumps explosive strength

Group	Trial	Mean jump height (cm) (± SD)	Effect size (d)	t-Test (p)	Mean flight time (ms) (± SD)	Effect size (d)	t-test (p)	Mean peak force (N) (± SD)	Effect size (d)	t-test (p)
VS (N = 22)	Pre	20.0 ± 3.0			402.9 ± 30.0			847.5 ± 248.0		
VS (N = 22)	Post	19.9 ± 3.5	0.05	0.65	400.1 ± 34.2	0.08	0.48	839.4 ± 278.4	0.03	0.47
SES (N = 8)	Pre	19.9 ± 4.0			400.3 ± 40.6			815.8 ± 243.4		
SES (N = 8)	Post	18.5 ± 3.4	0.37	0.05	389.0 ± 40.2	0.28	0.14	803.8 ± 249.7	0.49	0.42
VES (N = 7)	Pre	19.2 ± 2.6			395.1 ± 26.2			843.1 ± 304.2		
VES (N = 7)	Post	19.0 ± 2.7	0.09	0.75	392.6 ± 27.3	0.09	0.74	834.6 ± 312.0	−0.002	0.97

Table represents static jumps' explosive strength data from all groups: vibration stretching (VS), stretching only (SF) and vibration only (VF).
Reprinted from Kinser AM, Ramsey MW, O'Bryant HS et al (2008) Vibration and stretching effects on flexibility and explosive strength in young gymnasts. *Medicine and Science in Sports and Exercise* 40(1):133–140, with permission from

cating that future research may require a change from the stretch–vibration protocol using a longer duration of vibration than the 10-s period used by themselves and by Sands et al (2006). Future investigations should address the addition of vibration to stretching as a warm-up programme.

The purpose of the study by Wakeling et al (2002) was to identify how the lower extremity muscles minimize the soft-tissue resonance that occurs in response to pulsed and continuous mechanical vibration. In their study two hypotheses were tested: muscle activity increases the natural frequency to minimize resonance when the excitation frequency is close to the natural frequency of the soft tissues. The second hypothesis was how muscle activity would increase the damping to minimize resonance when the excitation frequency is close to the natural frequency of the soft tissues. Ten male (age 25.6 ± 1.2 years) and 10 female (age 23.1 ±) athletic subjects were tested, while standing on a vibration platform driven by a hydraulic actuator. Continuous vibrations and pulsed bursts of vibrations were presented, across the frequency range of 10–65 Hz and with peak-to-peak amplitude of the platform displacement of 5 mm. The test consisted of a cycle of 3 s of vibration followed by 3 s of no platform movement. During each vibration period, the frequency and amplitude of the platform vibration were kept constant. Frequencies of 10, 13.1, 17.1, 22.3, 29.1, 38.1, 49.7 and 65.0 Hz were tested. These eight frequencies were presented in a randomized block. The randomized block was then repeated five times so that the subject experienced a total of 40 periods of vibration in each test. Soft-tissue vibrations were measured with triaxial accelerometers, and muscle activity was measured by using surface electromyography from the quadriceps, hamstrings, tibialis anterior and triceps surae muscle groups. The measurements were taken with the subjects standing with a knee-flexion angle of 23°, which would mimic the knee posture at heel strike during running. The results demonstrate an elevated muscle activity in the EMG and an increased damping of vibration power which occurred when the frequency of the input was close to the natural frequency of each respective soft tissue. However, the natural frequency of the soft tissues did not change in a manner that correlated with the frequency of the input. The natural frequencies of the quadriceps, tibialis anterior and triceps surae range from 10 Hz for the relaxed condition to 50 Hz in a fully active state (Wakeling & Nigg 2001). The soft tissues are expected to resonate if the excitation frequency of a mechanical stimulus is close to the natural frequency of the soft tissues. It has been proposed that during walking and running the soft tissues of the lower extremity have a strategy of minimizing the soft-tissue vibrations (Nigg 1997). The body has a strategy of tuning muscle activity, in this case of the lower limb, in order to respond to the excitation frequency of the impact shock at heel strike during walking or running. It appears, as a result of this study, that soft-tissue damping may be the mechanism by which resonance is minimized at heel strike during running and the changes in frequency may have been a consequence of the altered muscle activity. Impact forces during heel–toe running typically have a major frequency component between 10 and 20 Hz. This frequency range spans the natural frequencies of the soft tissues measured in this study, which were 15 Hz. Thus there is potential for vibrations in the soft tissues to occur as a result of the impact forces. In order for the soft tissues to vibrate in such a manner they must have viscoelastic properties. During soft-tissue vibrations mechanical energy can be stored and returned from the elastic structures of the tendon and the attached cross-bridges. Damping of the vibrations results in a net dissipation of mechanical energy which can be absorbed by activated muscle.

Conclusion

These preliminary results offer convincing evidence that WBV has a role to play as a warm-up to ballistic weight-bearing high-impact sports, in which muscle length, temperature and resonance frequencies can have an impact on sporting achievement as well as playing a role in the reduction in the incidence of injury.

Exercise proposals: stretching section

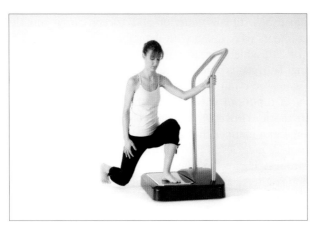

Figure 6.4 Stretching of quadriceps and iliopsoas muscles.

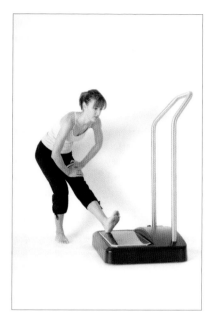

Figure 6.5 Stretching of hamstring muscles.

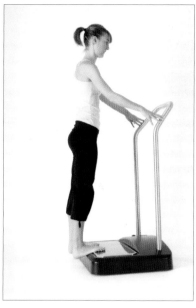

Figure 6.6 Stretching of gastrocnemius muscles.

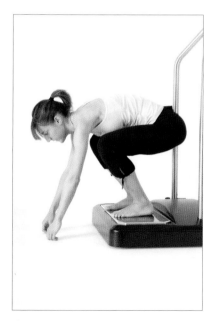

Figure 6.7 Stretching of soleus muscles.

References

Cardinale M, Bosco C (2003) The effects of vibration as an exercise intervention. *Exercise and Sport Sciences Reviews* 31:3–7.

Cardinale M, Lim J (2003) Electromyography activity of vastus lateralis muscle during whole body vibrations of different frequencies. *Journal of Strength & Conditioning Research* 17(3):621–624.

Issurin V, Liebermann DG, Tenenbaum G (1994) Effect of vibratory stimulation training on maximal force and flexibility. *Journal of Sports Sciences* 12:561–566.

Kerschan-Schindl K, Grampp S, Henk C (2001) Whole-body vibration exercise leads to alterations in muscle blood volume. *Clinical Physiology* 21:377–382.

Kinser AM, Ramsey MW, O'Bryant HS et al (2008) Vibration and stretching effects on flexibility and explosive strength in young gymnasts. *Medicine and Science in Sports and Exercise* 40(1):133–140.

Lycholat T (1990) *The Complete Book of Stretching*. Crosswood Press, Aylesbury.

Nazarov V, Zilinsky L (1984) Enhanced development of athletes strength abilities by means of biomechanical stimulation method. *Theory and Practice of Physical Culture Moscow* 10:28–30.

Nigg BM (1997) Impact forces in running. *Current Opinion in Orthopaedics* 8:43–47.

Sands WA, McNeal JR, Stone MH et al (2006) Flexibility enhancement with vibration: acute and long-term. *Medicine and Science in Sports and Exercise* 38:720–725.

Van den Tillaar R (2006) Will whole-body vibration training help increase the range of motion of the hamstrings? *Journal of Strength & Conditioning Research* 20(1):192–196.

Wakeling JM, Nigg BM (2001) Modification of soft tissue vibrations in the leg by muscular activity. *Journal of Applied Physiology* 90:412–420.

Wakeling JM, Bigg BM, Rozitis AI (2002) Muscle activity damps the soft tissue resonance that occurs in response to pulsed and continuous vibrations. *Journal of Applied Physiology* 93(3):1093–1103.

Wakeling J, Liphardt A, Nigg BM (2003) Muscle activity reduces soft-tissue resonance at heel-strike during walking. *Journal of Biomechanics* 36:1761–1769.

Appendix: **Synopsis of research into WBV**

Table 6.3 Synopsis of research into WBV, compiled by Martin Krause and Alfio Albasini

Researchers, names	Type of research	Dose	Exercise	Methodology	Outcome
Abercromby et al (2007), *Med Sci Sports Exerc* 39(10):1794–1800	Vertical forces to both feet vs upward forces to one leg at a time	30 Hz; 4 mm, 10 min	Slow unloaded squats	$n = 16$, comparative	Vertical forces to both feet simultaneously exceeds recommended daily vibration exposure (ISO 2631-1). Effects may be lower in half squats than full squats; and may be less in one legged loading.
Abercromby et al (2007), *Med Sci Sports Exerc* 39(9):1642–1650	Vertical vibration versus rotational vibration	30 Hz, 4 mm	Static and dynamic squatting	$n = 16$, comparative	EMG response in leg extensors was significantly greater in the rotational vibration group.
Annette et al (2005), NSCA conference presentation, 7 July University of Houston and University of Texas	Neuromuscular responses to two WBV modalities during dynamic squats	Power plate–vertical vibration 30 Hz, 4 mm: Vibraflex (rotates around an axis) at 30 Hz and 4 mm	Dynamic squat; stance 21.6 cm, 10–40° knee flexion; 4 s down and 4 s up	2×2 repeated measures (MANOVA), univariate ANOVAS and t-test (Sidak adjustment)	Vibraflex elicits greater response in the gastrocnemius (92 vs 49%), tibialis anterior (31 vs 16%), vastus lateralis (49 vs 32%), EMGrms in Vibraflex was greater than in PowerPlate in vastus lateralis (13%) and gastroc soleus (29%).

Table 6.3 Synopsis of research into WBV, compiled by Martin Krause and Alfio Albasini—cont'd

Researchers, names	Type of research	Dose	Exercise	Methodology	Outcome
Bautmans et al (2005), *BMC Geriatrics* 5:17	The feasibility of WBV in institutionalized elderly persons and its influence on muscle performance, balance and mobility	30–40 Hz, 2–5 mm, 3× per week, minimum 1 rest day between exercise	6 static exercises targeting lower limbs–exercise volume and intensity were increased based on overload principle	n = 24, nursing home patients, randomized control, static exercise ± WBV	Completion rate 96% with WBV and 86% controls. Training induced changes timed up-and-go and Tinetti-test were better for WBV ($p = 0.029$ and $p = 0.002$ resp.). Leg extensor work, power, explosive power, and maximal force, lower body flexibility improved significantly.
Baum et al (2007), *Int J Med Sci* 4:159–163	Efficiency of vibration exercise for glycaemic control in patients with type 2 diabetes	Vibrogym swinging platform, 2 mm, 30 Hz weeks 1–9, 35 Hz weeks 9–12, duration of single bout of exercise 30 s, 8 different exercises. Total duration was 20 min in last 3 weeks	Vibration, 3 days per week for 12 weeks, volume and intensity increased stepwise at 6 and 12 weeks; strength training 12 reps 70% 1RM, then 3 sets 10 reps at 80% 1RM for approx 45 min. Flexibility, group positions kept for 20 s, weeks 6–9 progression by 1 more set. Last 2 weeks, stretches for 30 s, total of 15 min	n = 40, randomized control, flexibility group, strength group vs vibration group	Decrease in systolic blood pressure in all interventions. No sign changes in endurance capacity. However, at 4 mmol lactate threshold heart rate was less for vibration group. Increase by 14% in max isometric torque in resistance training and vibration group. Small decrease in HbA1c values in vibration group potentially due to translocation of GLUT-4 to the sarcolemmal membrane which enhances glucose transport capacity.

Bazett-Jones et al (2008), *J Sports Sci Med* 7:144–150	WBV and countermovement jump	Power Plate	45 s, WBV at 2.16g (30 Hz, 2–4 mm), 2.80g (40 Hz, 2–4 mm), 4.87g (35 Hz, 4–6 mm), 5.83g (50 Hz, 4–6 mm)	n = 11, healthy males and females, random allocation of acceleration, with at least 2 days of rest between sessions	Women performed significantly better after 2.8g and 5.83g on CMJ (9.8 and 8.3%, resp). No change in men.
Belay et al (2008), *Spine* 33(5):E121–E131	Resistive simulated weight-bearing exercise with WBV reduces lumbar spine deconditioning in bed rest	Galileo, 19–26 Hz, amplitude 3.5–4 mm, 1.2–1.8g via elastic shoulder straps	Squats to 90° flexion, heel raises (with knees in extension), toe raises (knee extension and ankle dorsiflexion), each exercise >60 s, 10 reps explosive kicks at 10 s intervals (from near full hip and knee flexion). Vibration increased if subject could perform exercise for >100 s. Afternoon sessions were between 60 and 80% of static morning force	n = 20, randomized control, 8 weeks of strict bed rest with 6-month follow-up, after 8 weeks of bed rest, n = 1 attrition due to MRI phobia	Limited lumbar multifidus atrophy and atrophy did not persist in long term as in the control group, spinal lengthening and increases in disc area were reduced in the exercise group. Multifidus (MF) and erector spinae demonstrated contrasting relationships in CSA with MF increasing CSA with increased lordosis angle and disc height and only marginal correlation with spinal length, whereas LES increased CSA with spinal lengthening and increases in disc area but is unaffected by lordosis angle or disc height.

Table 6.3 Synopsis of research into WBV, compiled by Martin Krause and Alfio Albasini—cont'd

Researchers, names	Type of research	Dose	Exercise	Methodology	Outcome
Bogaerts et al (2007), *J Gerontol A Biol Sci Med Sci*, 62(6):630–635	1 year WBV on isometric and explosive muscle strength and muscle mass			Comparative, WBV ($n = 31$) vs fitness group ($n = 30$), vs sedentary ($n = 36$)	WBV training is as efficient as fitness training and therefore suggests it could prevent or reverse sarcopenia.
Bosco et al (n.d.) University of Rome	The influence of WBV on the mechanical behaviour of skeletal muscle	Galileo 2000, 26 Hz, acceleration 10 mm, acceleration 27 m/s², standing on toes, half-squat, feet rotated externally, single right leg 90° squat, single left leg 90° squat (for the last two positions subjects could maintain balance using a bar)	10 days, 5 sets of vertical sinusoidal vibrations lasting 90 s each, 40 s break between sets for a total of 10 min/day, every day 5 s was added until 2 min per position was reached. Total = WBV of 100 min at 2.7g = intensity of 200 drop jumps from 60 cm twice a week for 12 months (total time for drop jump is only 200 ms and the acceleration developed cannot reach 2.7g)	$n = 14$, physically active randomized control (handball and water polo players)	Increased height of best jump (1.6%, $p < 0.05$), mechanical power of best jump (3.1%, $p < 0.05$), average jumping height during 5 s (12%, $p < 0.01$). No change in CMJ potentially due to its larger angular displacement and slow stretching speed (3–6 rad/s) vs counter jump which has a faster stretch speed that is likely to enhance the gamma dynamic fusimotor response: • Increasing synchronization of motor units • Improvement in co-contraction of synergistic muscles? • Muscle spindles and Golgi tendon organ.

Reference	Title	Device / parameters	Protocol	Subjects	Results
Bosco et al (1999a), *Eur J Appl Physiol* 79:306–311	Influence of vibration on mechanical power and EMG activity in human arm flexor muscles	Galileo 2000, 30 Hz, 6 mm (acceleration 34 m/s²), vibrating dumbbell, with upper arms resting on plate in seated position	Static biceps curl, 5× 60 s, with 60 s rest in between. Total = 300 s = 600 elbow flexion moves at a load equal to 5% body mass = 3× per week with 50 reps each time would take 1 month	$n = 12$, international boxers, randomly assigned opposite arm as control	Enhanced muscle power and decreased EMG/power relationship, EMGrms activity increased up to more than twice baseline values during the activity.
Bosco et al (1999b), *Clin Physiol* 19(2):183–18	Adaptive responses of human skeletal muscle to vibration	Galileo 2000, 26 Hz, 10 mm, acceleration = 54 m/s²	WBV in one leg 100° flexion, 10 times 60 s, with 60 s rest in between. Total = 10 min WBV at $5.4g$ = 150 leg presses or half squats with extra loads (3× BW), × 2/week for 5 week	$n = 6$, national–level female volleyball players, leg randomly assigned	Shift to the right of the force–velocity curve similar to those observed after several weeks of heavy resistance training (Hakkinen & Komi 1985)

Table 6.3 Synopsis of research into WBV, compiled by Martin Krause and Alfio Albasini—cont'd

Researchers, names	Type of research	Dose	Exercise	Methodology	Outcome
Bosco et al (2000), *Eur J Appl Physiol* 81:449–454	Hormonal responses to WBV in men	Vertical sinusoidal	10× for 60 s, with 60 s rest between the vibration sets (a rest between the vibration sets lasting 6 min was allowed after five vibration sets)	Fourteen male subjects (mean age 25), non-randomized controlled	Significant increase in the plasma concentration of testosterone and GH, whereas cortisol levels decreased. An increase in the mechanical power output of the leg extensor muscles was observed with a reduction in EMGrms activity. Neuromuscular efficiency improved, as indicated by the decrease in the ratio between EMGrms and power. Jumping performance, which was measured using CMJ test, was also enhanced.
Bruyere et al (n.d.) conference presentation WHO	Controlled WBV to decrease fall risk and improve health-related quality of life in elderly patients	10 Hz 1st and 3rd series, 27 Hz 2nd and 4th series	6 weeks WBV, 4× 1 min, 3× per week, Galileo 900	n = 42, randomized control	Seven items of the SF-36 improved significantly: physical function (143%), pain (41%), vitality (60%), and general health (23%); also improvements in quality of walking (57%), equilibrium (77%), get up and go test (39%)

Reference	Study	Protocol	Subjects	Results
Bruyere et al (2005), *Arch Phys Med Rehab* 86:303–307	Controlled WBV to decrease fall risk and improve health-related quality of life in elderly patients. High-frequency WBV on balancing ability in older women	10 Hz 1st and 3rd session, 26 Hz at 2nd and 4th session, peak to peak 30 and 7 mm respectively. Side alternating 20 Hz, 3 min/day, 3 days/week for 3 months	6 weeks WBV, 4× 1 min, 3× per week, Galileo 900	$n = 42$, randomized control, $n = 69$	Body balance improved 3.5% ± 2.1, TUG decreased by 11.0 ± 8.6, improvements in eight of nine items in SF-36. Enhanced stability in movement velocity ($p < 0.01$), maximum point excursion ($p < 0.01$), and directional control ($p < 0.05$).
Cheug et al (2007), *Arch Phys Med Rehab* 88(7):852–857	High-frequency WBV on balancing ability in older women	Side alternating 20 Hz, 3 min/day, 3 days/week for 3 months		$n = 69$, randomized control	Enhanced stability in movement velocity ($p < 0.01$), maximum point excursion ($p < 0.01$), and directional control ($p < 0.05$).
Cardinale (2002), PhD thesis	Effect of vibration on human performance and hormonal profile	6–10 mm peak to peak, 26–30 Hz	1) 10 days 2) 5 min static position in professional volleyball players	$n = 62$, physically active and involved in regular exercise 1) Chronic exposure for 10/7 ($n = 14$) 2) Acute effects of vibration on force/velocity relationship ($n = 6$)	1) Average jumping height during 5 s continuous jumping improved by 11.5%; no change to counter-jump; no change in muscle bulk, suggesting neural effect, particularly as stiffness increased probably due to Ia loop feedback

Table 6.3 Synopsis of research into WBV, compiled by Martin Krause and Alfio Albasini—cont'd

Researchers, names	Type of research	Dose	Exercise	Methodology	Outcome
				3) Dumbbell vibration in boxers ($n = 12$) 4) Verify acute hormonal response, 7 min for well-trained handball players ($n = 14$) 5) Hormonal response but total 10 mins, divided in two sets of five subsets lasting 1 min each, 6 min rest between sets 6) Fatiguing exercises with/without WBV	2) Shift of force/power and power/velocity relationship to the right ($p < 0.05$)–neural as there was not increase in cross-sectional area 3) Also shown to increase (by 13%) arm flexor mechanical power using a similar protocol (EMGrms increase by 200%) 4) Vertical jumping ability declined together with increases in serum testosterone and serum cortisol concentrations, suggesting 7 min protocol as a stressful treatment 5) Testosterone levels improved by 7%, growth hormone levels increased 460%, and cortisol reduced by 32%, vertical jump increased 4%, leg press increased 7%, EMG knee extensors decreased 10%

6) Dynamic exercise with superimposed WBV increased average power output by 8%, whereas arm action was 14% higher due to large motor unit recruitment.

Reference	Aim / measure	Vibration device / parameters	Protocol	Subjects / method	Results
Cardinale et al (2005), *Br J Sports Med* 39:585–589				Literature review	Not superior to traditional training methods in highly trained athletes. More appropriate for sedentary and elderly.
Cardinale et al (2007), *Med Sci Sports Exerc* 39(4);694–700	Gastrocnemius medialis (GM) and vastus lateralis (VL) oxygenation (TOI)	30, 40 and 50 Hz Fitwave	Static squatting for 110 s	$n = 20$, randomized crossover design, (10 sedentary, 10 athletes)	TOI of VL decreased by 2.8% at 90 s in control, decreased by 3.3% at 110 s at 30 Hz; TOI of VL decreased by 2.1 and 3.0% at 110 s at 40 and 50 Hz, respectively; GM TOI decreased by 3.2% at 60 s, 4.1% at 90 s and 4.3% in control, and by 5.5% at 110 s at 30 Hz. Therefore, not a significant difference in WBV compared with controls.
Cochrane et al (2008), *J Sci Med Sport* 11(6):527–534	Acute effects of vibration exercise on concentric muscular characteristics	Electric power dumbbell, 26 Hz, amplitude 3 mm, 30 s exposure at five different shoulder positions		$n = 12$, comparative between vibration, arm cranking (25 W) and control on maximal prone bench pull capacity	Vibration increased concentric peak power 4.8% vs increase by 3% for cranking over control. No change in EMG.

Table 6.3 Synopsis of research into WBV, compiled by Martin Krause and Alfio Albasini—cont'd

Researchers, names	Type of research	Dose	Exercise	Methodology	Outcome
Da Silva et al (2007), *J Strength Cond Res* 21(2):470–475	Influence of vibration training on energy expenditure in active men		Five sets of 10 reps, 2-min recovery between sets, half squats	$n = 17$, comparative, half-squat with/without WBV, random sequence order	Energy expenditure and perceived exertion were significantly greater with WBV.
De Ruiter et al (2003), *Eur J Appl Physiol* 90:595–600	The effects of 11 weeks' WBV training on jump height, contractile properties and activation of human knee extensors	30 Hz, 8 mm amplitude	3× per week and stood bare-foot with a 110° knee angle on a vibration platform. Not progressive training as required for progressive overload training	10 subjects belonging to the experimental group trained, another 10 subjects were in the control group	Quadriceps femoris isometric muscle force [105.4 (6.2)%, 99.9 (2.0)%; $p = 0.69$], voluntary activation [107.1 (6.0)%, 101.1 (2.3)%; $p = 0.55$] and maximal rate of voluntary force rise [95.4 (6.0)%, 103.3 (7.7)%; $p = 0.57$] did not improve. The maximal rate of force rise during electrical stimulation was increased [102.3 (4.5)%, 123.6 (7.5)%; $p = 0.02$]. CMJ height was not affected by WBV [103.7 (1.8)%, 103.0 (2.8)%; $p = 0.71$].

Reference	Aim	Frequency	Protocol	Subjects	Results
Delecluse et al (2003), *Med Sci Sports Exerc* 35(6):1033–1041	Strength increase after WBV compared with resistance training	35–40 Hz, 2.28–5.09g	Static and dynamic knee extensor exercises, 3× per week. Resistance training (RES) group performed 10–20 RM	$n = 67$, randomized control, untrained females, comparative WBV vs RES versus placebo (PL)	Isometric and dynamic knee-extensor strength increased significantly ($p < 0.001$) in both the WBV group (16.6 ± 10.8%; 9.0 ± 3.2%) and the RES group (14.4 ± 5.3%; 7.0 ± 6.2%), respectively, whereas the PL and CO groups showed no significant ($p > 0.05$) increase. CMJ height enhanced significantly ($p < 0.001$) in the WBV group (7.6 ± 4.3%) only. There was no effect of any of the interventions on maximal speed of movement, as measured by means of ballistic tests.
Delecluse et al (2005), *Int J Sports Med* 26:662–668	Effects of WBV on muscle strength and sprint performance in sprint-trained athletes	35–40 Hz, 1.7–2.5 mm Power Plate	5 weeks, unloaded static and dynamic leg exercises	$n = 20$, randomized control	Specific WBV protocol had no surplus value upon the conventional training programme to improve speed strength performance in sprint-trained athletes
Di Loreto et al (2004), *J Endocrinol Invest* 27:323–327	Effects of WBV exercise on the endocrine system of healthy men	30 Hz	Volunteers were studied on two occasions before and after standing for 25 min on a ground	10 healthy men [age 39 ± 3, body mass index (BMI) of 23.5 ± 0.5 kg/m², mean ± SEM]	Vibration slightly reduced plasma glucose (30 min: vibration 4.59 ± 0.21, control 4.74 ± 0.22 mM, $p = 0.049$) and increased plasma norepinephrine concentrations

Table 6.3 Synopsis of research into WBV, compiled by Martin Krause and Alfio Albasini—cont'd

Researchers, names	Type of research	Dose	Exercise	Methodology	Outcome
			plate in the absence (control) or in the presence (vibration)		60 min: vibration 1.29 ± 0.18, control 1.01 ± 0.07 nM, ($p = 0.038$), but did not change the circulating concentrations of other hormones (insulin, cortisol, epinephrine, GH, IGF-1, free and total testosterone.
Erskine et al (2007), *Clin Physiol Funct Imaging* 27(4):242–248	Acute hormonal response to WBV	30 Hz, 3.5g, 10 min	10 sets of half isometric squats for 1 min, with 1 min rest between sets	$n = 7$, comparative control	Acute reduction in MVC, which recovered after 24 hours. No change in testosterone or cortisol concentration.
Fagnani et al (2006), *Am J Phys Med Rehab* 85:956–962	Muscle performance and flexibility in female athletes		8-week protocol, 3 days per week vertical vibration platform	$n = 26$, randomized control, female athletes	Improved maximal knee extension strength, CMJ and flexibility.
Feltham et al (2006), *J Biomechanics* 39:2850–2856	Changes in joint stability with muscle contraction measured from transmission of mechanical vibration	Mechanical vibration at 45, 50 and 55 Hz to styloid process of radius and distal end of metacarpal bone of index finger		$n = 10$	Gain was calculated at five force levels ranging from 5 to 25% of Max grip force (MF) and a trend for 15% MF and higher at 55 Hz; transfer function gain increases with muscle co-contraction of antagonist muscles and most likely due to increased joint stiffness.

Fontana et al (2005), *Aust J Physiol* 51:259–263	The effect of weight-bearing exercise with low-frequency, WBV on lumbosacral proprioception: a pilot study on normal subjects	18 Hz (Rittweger et al 2002), feet 25 cm apart, pelvis rotated forward and backward. Galileo 2000	Single 5-min static semi-squat	$n = 25$, randomized control, young healthy	Experimental group demonstrated 39% improvement in re-positioning accuracy (mean 0.78°).
Garataachea et al (2007), *J Strength Cond Res* 21(2):594–598	Effects of movement velocity during squatting on energy expenditure and substrate utilization in WBV	30 Hz, 4 mm, 3 min, with additional load of 30% body weight	Three squatting exercises in execution frequency cycles of 6, 4 and 2 s to 90°	$n = 9$, comparative, WBV vs non WBV, two-way ANOVA	Squatting at greater frequency helps to maximize energy expenditure during exercise with/ without vibration and therefore cycle time duration must be controlled when prescribing WBV.
Gusi et al (2006), *BMC Musculoskeletal Disorders*; 7(92):1–8	Low-frequency vibratory exercise reduces the risk of bone fracture more than walking	Lower than 20 Hz	Three sessions per week for 8 months, six bouts of 1 min (12.6 Hz, 3 cm amplitude, 60° knee flexion)	$n = 28$, randomized control trial, untrained postmenopausal healthy women (average age 66)	BMD femoral neck increased 4.3% more than walking group. BMD lumbar spine unaltered in both groups. Balance improved in WBV by 29%.

Table 6.3 Synopsis of research into WBV, compiled by Martin Krause and Alfio Albasini—cont'd

Researchers, names	Type of research	Dose	Exercise	Methodology	Outcome
Haas et al (2006), *NeuroRehabilitation* 21:29–36	The effects of random WBV on motor symptoms in Parkinson's disease	ZEPTORmed system, Scisens, Germany. 6 Hz, amplitude 3 mm	Five series of WBV, 60 s each	$n = 68$, randomized crossover design	Well tolerated. UPDRS motor score reduced by 5.2 and 4.8 representing reductions of 16.8 and 14.7%. Highest improvements in tremor and rigidity (25 and 24%). Gait and posture items show 15% improvement. Bradykinesia scores were reduced by 12%.
Hazell et al (2007), *Appl Physiol Nutr Metab* 32(6):1156–1163	The effects of WBV on upper and lower body EMG during static and dynamic contractions	Vertically oscillating platform—determination of optimal WBV stimulus (frequency × amplitude), 2 and 4 mm at 25, 30, 35, 40 and 45 Hz	Static semi-squat, and dynamic squat	$n = 10$, using EMG RMS frequencies as %MVC	Higher WBV amplitude (4 mm) and frequencies (35, 40, 45 Hz) resulted in greatest increases in EMG activity (increase VL by 2.9–6.7% in static and 3.7–8.7% in dynamic conditions).
Hopkins et al (2007), *Int J Sports Med*, Sep 18	Changes in peroneus longus activation following ankle inversion perturbation after WBV			$n = 22$, two-way ANOVAs comparison over three time intervals	No changes.

Iwamato et al (2005), *Aging Clin Exp Res* 17(2):157–63	Effects of WBV on lumbar bone mineral density and low back pain in post-menopausal osteoporotic women treated with alendronate	20 Hz, once per week, 4 min, Galileo system, lasting 12 months	n = 50, randomized to alendronate ± WBV, (25 each group)	WBV using Galileo appears to be useful for LBP, probably by relaxing the back muscles. No differences in BMD, neither N-terminal, telopeptides type I collagen nor serum alkaline phosphatase (ALP), were seen.
Issurin & Tenenbaum (1999), *J Sports Sci* 17:177–182	Acute and residual effects of vibratory stimulation on explosive strength in elite and amateur athletes	44 Hz, acceleration 30 m/s^2	Vibratory stimulation during biceps curl, three sets: 8–10 repetition biceps curls low to medium load (20–40% BW), then 3–5 attempts at increasing weight. A weight of 65–70% 1RM was selected. Two series of exercises with 8–15 min recovery. Period of rest between sets was 2–3 min	n = 14 elite and n = 14 amateur athletes with/without vibration in random sequence of exercises	Increase by 30.1 and 29.8 W (10.4 and 10.2%) in max and mean power in elite athletes, 20 and 25.9 W (7.9 and 10.7%) in amateur athletes. Vibratory stimulation resulted in an insignificant residual effect.

Table 6.3 Synopsis of research into WBV, compiled by Martin Krause and Alfio Albasini—cont'd

Researchers, names	Type of research	Dose	Exercise	Methodology	Outcome
Judex et al (2007), *J Biomechanics* 40:1333–1339	Low-magnitude mechanical signals that stimulate bone formation in ovariectomized rat are dependent on the applied frequency but not strain magnitude	45 vs 90 Hz, 10 min per day		$n = 12$, comparative	Bone morphology at 90 Hz significantly greater trabecular volume (22 and 25%) and thicker trabecular (11 and 12%) over controls of 45 Hz in epiphysis of distal femur, despite strain rates and magnitudes being significantly lower at 90 than at 45 Hz.
Kawanabe et al (2007), *Keio J Med* 56(1):28–33	Effect of WBV exercise and muscle strengthening, balance, and walking exercises on walking ability in the elderly	12–20 Hz, 4 mins, once per week for 2 months, Galileo 2000	Standing on both legs with bent knees and hips	$n = 67$ elderly non-randomized active ± WBV	Walking speed (−14.9%), step length (+6.5%), maximum standing time on one leg (right +65%, left +88.4%) improved significantly in WBV + exercise group. No serious adverse events occurred during the study period.
Kemertzis et al (2008), *Med Sci Sports Exerc* 40(11), 1977–1983	Ankle flexors produce peak torque at longer muscle lengths after WBV	26 Hz, 5 × 1 min Galileo 900	Passive ankle stretch of the plantar flexors at end of range, followed by the same stretch with superimposed WBV	$n = 20$ young males; between treatment and within treatment outcomes were assessed using MANOVA	No change in the ROM; significant 7.1° shift in the angle of peak plantar flexor torque production corresponding with longer muscle lengths; some DOMS was experienced.

Kinser et al (2008), *J Athletic Training* 41(3):286–293	Vibration and stretching effects on flexibility and explosive strength in young gymnasts	30 Hz, 2 mm amplitude vibration box (vertical loaded/ cyclic manner)	10 s vibration-stretching at four different sites (quads, hamies hamstrings, calves, adductors), 5 s rest between stretches, four repetitions each	$n = 22$ young female athletes (age = 11.3 ± 2.6 years), randomized four groups–flexibility group and explosive strength group consisting of stretching only, vibration only	Simultaneous stretching and vibration may greatly increase flexibility while not altering explosive strength.
Mahieu et al (2006), *J Athletic Training* 41(3):286–293	Improving strength and posture control in young skiers: WBV versus equivalent resistance training	WBV platform Fitvibe	Squatting, deep squatting, wide stance squatting, 1-legged squatting, calf raises, skiing movements, jumps onto the plate, and light jumping. 3× 30 min per week. Week 1 training: three exercises 30 s each, 60 s rest. Training intensity increased over 6/52 with	$n = 33$, randomized control, Belgian competitive skiers, control group had significantly lower knee torque and ankle torque prior to training. Knee • Extension 92.35 vs 78.5 • Flexion 66.35 vs 53.33	Significant (statistical and functional) difference in high box test and plantar flexion torque at 30°/s.

Table 6.3 Synopsis of research into WBV, compiled by Martin Krause and Alfio Albasini—cont'd

Researchers, names	Type of research	Dose	Exercise	Methodology	Outcome
			increased amplitude 2–4 mm and increased frequency 24–28 Hz. Also increased duration and number of repetitions. Week 6 training: four exercises, 250 s total duration, 60 s rest. Resistance training group had exactly same protocol minus the WBV	Ankle • Extension 70.82 vs 60.62 • Flexion 11.2 vs 7.76	
Maloney-Hinds et al (2008), *Med Sci Monit* 14(3):CR112–116	The effect of 30 Hz vs 50 Hz passive vibration and duration of vibration on skin blood flow in the arm	30 vs 50 Hz to the arms for 10 min	Passive vibration	Randomized 30 or 50 Hz for $n = 18$ and both frequencies for $n = 7$	5 min of 30 and 50 Hz vibration produced significant increases in skin blood flow, 50 Hz appeared to be more beneficial as there was not vasoconstriction during the recovery period.
Mark et al–conference presentation	Metabolic and cardiovascular responses during WBV–a pilot study	Increasing vibration challenge by varying frequency (19.6 Hz stages 2 and 4; 27.8 Hz stages 1 and 3) of WBV and foot placement (which	3-min stages of vibration followed by 3 min rest	$n = 6$	Moderate intensity WBV results in increased femoral artery blood flow (2–4 mL/min); no change in MAP or in femoral artery diameter. Significantly high variable psychological stress (effort perception)

Reference	Title	Method	Measure	Sample	Results
Mileva et al (2006), *Med Sci Sports Exerc* 38(7):1317–1328	Acute effects of a vibration-like stimulus during knee extension exercise	10 Hz superimposed stimulus to knee extension at 35 (low) and 70% (high intensity), Vibrex system, Exoscience, Technogym Ltd UK; varies displacement amplitude and gravitational load using Galileo 2000	1RM 35% and 70% MVC	$n = 9$, four trials of 1RM	Superimposed 10 Hz at 35%MVC speed up the rate of vastus lateralis deoxygenation, modest improvements in peak torque
Moezy et al (2008), *Br J Sports Med*, Jan 8	WBVT vs conventional training on proprioception and knee stability after ACL reconstruction			$n = 20$, comparative	WBVT improved proprioception and balance in ACL reconstructed athletes.
Moran et al (2007), *Med Sci Sports Exerc* 39(3):526–533	Effect of vibration training in 70%MVC dynamic biceps curl	65 Hz, 1.2 mm strapped over biceps tendon	1RM 70%MVC biceps curl	$n = 14$, crossover design	No change mean angular velocity, peak angular velocity, mean moment, peak moment, mean power, peak power.

Table 6.3 Synopsis of research into WBV, compiled by Martin Krause and Alfio Albasini—cont'd

Researchers, names	Type of research	Dose	Exercise	Methodology	Outcome
Mulder et al (2007), *J Electromyogr Kines* 19(2):208–218	High-density surface EMG, CNS and PNS 8 weeks' bed rest with/without resistive vibration exercise	18 Hz	Supine lying 10 'explosive' squats, 10 s rest a.m. Progressive training based on 'overload' principle, adjusted weekly, 10–17 repetitions a.m. (60–100 s) and 70%MVC p.m. (60 s)	Comparative, randomized, control	Prevented bed rest atrophy and improved maximal amplitude on EMG by 30% from day 10 onwards; however, this was task specific at the peripheral motor unit site and hence did not prevent task-non-specific loss of function.
Nishihira et al (2002), *Adv Exerc Sports Physiol* 8(4):83–86	Effect of WBV stimulus and voluntary contraction on motoneurone pool	25 Hz, static knee angle 100–120°	Three sets of 3 min, 10-min break between sets, using Galileo 2000	$n = 17$, EMG of soleus muscle and H-reflex	H-reflex increased suggestive an increase in excitability of the motor neurone pool
Rittweger et al (2000), *Clin Physiol* 20(2):134–142	Acute physiological effects of exhaustive WBV exercise in man	26 Hz, feet 15 cm from rotation axis, vibration amplitude 1.05 cm, peak acceleration 147 m/s² = 15g	Squatting + additional load 40% body weight, 3 s down, 3 s up	$n = 37$	Borg scale perceived exertion 18, HR 128 beats/min, blood pressure 132/52, lactate 3.5 mM, oxygen 48.8% of max. vol, knee extension reduced by 9.2%, jump height reduced by 9.2%, jump height 9.1%, and decreased mEMG was attenuated.

Rittweger et al (2001), *Eur J Apl Physiol* 86:169–173	Oxygen uptake during WBV exercise: comparison with squatting as a slow voluntary movement	26 Hz, 6 mm, feet 24 cm apart, (approx 18*g* based on 30 Hz, acceleration	3 min squatting in cycles of 6 s, simple standing, squatting with an additional 35% body weight load for females and 40% load for males	$n = 12$	Vibration elicits a metabolic muscular response and therefore is not a passive form of exercise. Oxygen consumption increased 4.5 mL/min/kg. Using oxygen at 20.9 J/mL = 1.6 W (kg body mass). Walking speed at 0.4 m/s requires 2.3 mL/min/kg and therefore WBV is metabolically comparable to walking.
Rittweger et al (2002a), *Spine* 27(17):1892–1834	Treatment of chronic low back pain with lumbar extension and WBV exercise	18 Hz, 6 mm, 4 min in beginning and gradually increased to 7 min	18 exercise units were performed within 12 weeks, two units in first 6 weeks and then one unit per week thereafter, Galileo 2000, in static slight knee flexion, bending in frontal and saggital plane and rotating in the horizontal plane, 5 kg was added to the shoulders in later sessions	$n = 60$, randomized control, WBV vs back extension exercises	Significant reduction in pain sensation and pain-related disability observed in both groups.

Table 6.3 Synopsis of research into WBV, compiled by Martin Krause and Alfio Albasini—cont'd

Researchers, names	Type of research	Dose	Exercise	Methodology	Outcome
Rittweger et al (2002b), Int J Sports Med 23:428–432	Oxygen uptake in WBV–influence of frequency, amplitude and external load	18–34 Hz, 5 mm, addition of 40% lean body mass attached to waist and later shoulders		$n = 10$ changing frequencies, $n = 8$ changing amplitude	Vibration amplitude of 5 mm a linear increase in oxygen consumption from 18 to 34 Hz; at 26 Hz the oxygen consumption increased more than proportionally with amplitudes from 2.5 to 7.5 mm. Addition of loads increased the oxygen consumption significantly.
Rittweger et al (2003), Clin Physiol Funct Imaging 23(2):81–86	The neuromuscular effects of hard squatting with or without WBV	26 Hz (used because below 20 Hz induces relaxation; whereas above 50 Hz can induce severe muscle damage), 6 mm (12 mm from top to bottom)	Galileo 2000 prototype, 0–90° knee flexion, plus 40% lean body mass at hips, 3 s down and 3 s up, exercise until exhaustion	$n = 19$, randomized cross-over study, ANOVA	EMG median frequency increased over VL and was greater after WBV, attenuation of stretch reflex amplitude suggesting CNS recruitment, and spinal reflex pathways
Roelants et al (2004a), J Am Geriatr Soc 52(6):901–908	WBV training increases strength and speed of movement in older women	35–40 Hz 2.5–5.0 mm Power Plate. Total duration 5–30 min at the end of training	24 weeks WBV, unloaded static and dynamic knee extensor exercises	$n = 89$, randomized control, postmenopausal women, WBV, resistance training, control	Isometric and dynamic knee extensor strength increased in WBV (15 ± 2.1 and $16.1 \pm 3.1\%$) and resistance training (18.4 ± 2.8 and $13.9 \pm 2.7\%$ groups; $p = 0.558$). CMJ increased sign in WBV

Reference	Aim	Protocol	Study design	Study group	Results
					(19.4 ± 2.8%) and resistance training (12.9 ± 2.9%). Most effects within 12 weeks. $n = 6$ left the resistance training group due to anterior knee pain vs 1 in WBV group.
Roelants et al (2004b), Int J Sports Med 25(1):1–5	Effects of 24 weeks of WBV on body composition in untrained females	35–40 Hz 2.5–5.0 mm Power Plate. Total duration 5–30 min at the end of training	Unloaded static and dynamic exercises 3× weekly	$n = 48$, comparative WBV training vs fitness training, vs control, elderly women	Fat-free mass increased in WBV group only (+2.2%). Significant increases in strength in WBV 24.4 ± 5.1% and training group 16.5 ± 1.7%.
Rubin et al (2001), FASEB 15:2225–2229	Ability of extremely low-magnitude, high-frequency mechanical signals to restore anabolic bone cell activity inhibited by disuse	10 min per day at 90 Hz, 0.25g peak to peak for 28 days	Daily exposure to vibration vs disuse	Comparative six different groups	Bone formation rate (BFR) in the proximal tibia in the vibration group compared with the other group increased +97%.
Rubin et al (2003), Spine 28:2621–2627	Determine the degree of transmissibility of high-frequency low-magnitude mechanical signals, delivered through plantar surface of the foot to the hip and spine	Transcutaneous pins were placed in spinous process of L4 and greater trochanter of the femur of six volunteers. Standing on an oscillating platform	Vibration data were recorded at 2-Hz intervals beginning at 15 Hz and ending at 30 Hz	The participants were standing in three different postures: • Erect with knee extended and locked • Relaxed with knees straight • Knees flexed at 20°	With subjects standing erect, transmissibility at the hip exceeded 100% at 20 Hz. At more than 25 Hz transmissibility decreased to 80% at the hip and spine in relaxed stance, transmission decreased to 60% with 20° of knee flexion

Table 6.3 Synopsis of research into WBV, compiled by Martin Krause and Alfio Albasini—cont'd

Researchers, names	Type of research	Dose	Exercise	Methodology	Outcome
		data were collected from accelerometers fixed to the pins while a platform vibrated			
Rubin et al (2004), *J Bone Miner Res* 19:343–351	Bone mineral density	Two 10-min treatments, low magnitude 2.0g peak to peak, 30 Hz vertical acceleration for 1 year	Each day vibration just standing	$n = 70$, randomized, double-blind and placebo-controlled trial of postmenopausal women	Treatment group demonstrated an improvement of 2.17% in the femoral neck and 1.5% in the lumbar spine.
Rubin et al (2005), *Gene* 367:1–16	Molecular pathways mediating mechanical signalling in bone	Review considers the mechanical factors generated by loading in the skeleton, including strain, stress and pressure. Mechanosensitive cells which recognize these forces in the skeleton are reviewed. The identity of the mechanoreceptors is			

Rubin et al (2007), *Proc Natl Acad Sci USA* 104(45): 17879–17884	Adipogenesis is inhibited by brief daily exposure to high-frequency, extremely low-magnitude mechanical signals	5 days per week, 15 min, 90 Hz, 0.2g	15 weeks of brief daily exposure to vibration, vs walking	$n = 40$, comparative, mice	Inhibition of adipogenesis by 27%, reduced non-esterified free fatty acids and triglycerides by 43 and 39%. Over 9 weeks fat production was suppressed by 22% in C3HB6-6T accelerated age-related mice. Mesenchymal stem cell differentiation into adipocytes reduced by 19%.
Sands et al (2000) *Med Sci Sports Exerc* 38(4):720–725	Flexibility enhanced with vibration: acute and long term	30 Hz 2 mm displacement box	Stretching protocol over 4 weeks, 5 days/week, in forward/rear splits for calf and quads, 10 secs stretch, 50 secs off repeated four times which equaled 1 min of fatal stretching	$n = 10$, randomized young males gymnasts (age = 10.1 ± 1.5 yrs)	Promising means of attaining ROM beyond that achieved by static stretching in highly trained gymnasts.

Table 6.3 Synopsis of research into WBV, compiled by Martin Krause and Alfio Albasini—cont'd

Researchers, names	Type of research	Dose	Exercise	Methodology	Outcome
Savelberg et al (2007), *J Strength Cond Res* 21(2):589–593	WBV increase in muscle length results in muscle strength		Isometric knee extension	$n = 28$, randomized four groups, each group received 4/52 of WBV at one of three different frequencies (20, 27, 34 Hz) or one of two different lengths of knee extensors	Weaker subjects responded better (10–50% increase strength). Training at shorter lengths resulted in optimal angle shifts to greater lengths in both stronger and weaker subjects.
Spitzpfeil et al (2006), *J Biochemanics* 39(Suppl 1):S196, 5931	Mechanical impacts to the human body by different vibration training devices	Galileo 2000 vs Power Plate, 25, 30, 35, 40, 50 Hz; 0, 60, 80% body weight, knee angle 110° and 150°	15 s	$n = 8$, randomized	Acceleration to head by Power Plate was 02–06g which was sign higher than Galileo 2000 of 01–02g
Stewart et al (2004), *Am J Physiol Regul Integr Comp Physiol* 288(3):R623–R629	Plantar vibration improves leg fluid flow in perimenopausal women	0, 15, 45 Hz, at 35° tilt, 0.2g, 0.2 m^2	Passive tilt at 35° from horizontal	$n = 18$ perimenopausal women	Enhanced peripheral and systemic blood flow (25–35%), improved lymphatic flow and better venous drainage. Postulated this would be necessary for preventing osteopenia due to bone orthostasis.

Stewart et al (2007), *J Sci Med Sport* 12(1):50–53	Differential effects of WBV durations on knee extensor strength	Galileo 26 Hz, 4 mm, 2, 4 or 6 min	Static?	n = 12, comparative	2 min increased peak torque by 3.8%, 4 and 6 min decreased peak torque by −2.7 and −6%, respectively
Suhr et al (2006) *J Biomechanics* 39(Suppl 1) S196, 5174	Short-term vibration stimuli during intensive cycling performance on angiogenesis	30 Hz, 4-mm amplitude	90 min cycling	n = 12, cycling in normobaric hypoxia, and normoxia with/ without vibration, altitude of 2400 m, four weekly training sessions at weekly intervals in randomized order	Vibration significantly increased vascular endothelial growth factor (VEGF).
Thompson et al (2007), *Clin Neurophysiol* 118(11):2456–2467	Effect of bilateral Achilles vibration on posture	30 s of tendon vibration	Static?	n = 12, comparative; before, during, 5 and 25 s after vibration	Over and under-correction of initial position.
Tihanyi et al (2007), *Clin Rehabil* 21(9):782–793	WBV and strength after stroke	20 Hz, 5 mm, 6× 1 min	Static	n = 16, randomized control	Isometric and knee extensor torque increase by 36.6% and 22.2 respectively

Table 6.3 Synopsis of research into WBV, compiled by Martin Krause and Alfio Albasini—cont'd

Researchers, names	Type of research	Dose	Exercise	Methodology	Outcome
Torvinen et al (2002a), *Clin Physiol Funct Imaging* 22:145–152	Effect of a vibration exposure on muscular performance and body balance	4 min, feet 0.28 m from centre of platform, 15 Hz 1st minute, 20 Hz 2nd minute, 25 Hz 3rd minute, 30 Hz last minute, peak-to-peak amplitude 10 mm, acceleration was 3.5g at 15 Hz, 6.5g at 20 Hz, 10g at 25 Hz, 14g at 30 Hz	Repeated 4× multidirectional movement on platform—light squatting (0–10 s), standing in erect posture (10–20 s), standing in relaxed posture (20–30 s), light jumping (30–40 s), alternating body weight one leg to the other (40–50 s), and standing on heels (50–60 s)	$n = 16$, randomized crossover study	2.5% net benefit in jump height ($p = 0.019$), 3.2% benefit in isometric strength ($p = 0.020$), 15.7% improvement in body balance ($p = 0.049$) 2 min after WBV.
Torvinen et al (2002b), *Med Sci Sports Exerc* 34(9):1523–1528	Effect of 4-month vertical WBV on performance and balance	Vertical WBV, Kuntotary, Erka Oy, Finland. First 2 weeks, 25 Hz for 1 min, then 30 Hz for another minute. Next 1.5 months,	4 months, 4 min/day 3–5× per week, 4× 60 s, light squatting (0–10 s), standing in the erect position (10–20 s), standing relaxed knees slightly	Randomized controlled, young healthy non-athletic adults, $n = 56$, $n = 4$ dropout ($n = 2$ in WBV unrelated to training regimen)	No direct influence on body balance, vertical jump improved 2 cm (10.2% improvement) at 2 months, 2.5 cm improvement in vertical jump (8.5% increase) at 4 months. Isometric strength increase by 11.2 kg at 2 months

Reference	Aim	Protocol	Exercise	Subjects	Results
					(3.7% net benefit). No change in shuttle tests.
Van den Tillaar (2006), *J Strength Cond Res* 20(1):192–196	Will WBV training help increase the range of motion of the hamstrings?	3 min at 25 Hz/60 s + 30 Hz/60 s + 35 Hz/60 s. Remaining 2 months, 4 min at 25 Hz/60 s + 30 Hz/60 s + 35 Hz/60 s + 40 Hz/60 s. Acceleration 2.5g at 25 Hz, 3.6g at 30 Hz, 4.9g at 35 Hz, and 6.4g at 40 Hz	flexed (20–30 s), light jumping (30–40 s), alternating the body weight one leg to the other (40–50 s), standing on the heels (50–60 s)	Repeated measures ANCOVA, $n = 19$ (10 in WBV and 9 controls) randomly allocated men and women	Significant increases in hamstring flexibility. WBV group showed a significant increase (30%) in ROM compared with 14% for controls.
Van Nes et al (2004), *Am J Phys Med Rehab* 83(11):867–873	Short-term effects of WBV on postural control in unilateral chronic stroke patients: preliminary evidence	Commercial platform, 30 Hz, 3-mm amplitude	4× 45 s WBV in standing	$n = 23$, chronic stroke patients	Reduction in root mean square centre-of-pressure velocity in anterior–posterior direction with eyes shut, increase in weight shifting speed, precision remained constant. No adverse side-effects observed.

Table 6.3 Synopsis of research into WBV, compiled by Martin Krause and Alfio Albasini—cont'd

Researchers, names	Type of research	Dose	Exercise	Methodology	Outcome
Verschueren et al (2004), *J Bone Miner Res* 19(3):352–359	Effect of 6-month WBV training on hip density, muscle strength, and postural control in postmenopausal women: a randomized controlled pilot study	35–40 Hz, 2.28–5.09g	3× weekly for 24 weeks. WBV group performed static and dynamic knee extensor exercises; Resistance group started with low (20RM) to high (8RM) resistance. Control group, no exercise	n = 70, randomized controlled, WBV vs resistance training	No vibration-related side-effects. WBV improved isometric and dynamic muscle strength (+15 and +16%, respectively). Increases in BMD of hip (+0.93%); no change of BMD observed in resistance training group.
von der Heide et al (2004), Dept Gynecology and Obstetrics, George-August-University, Gottingen, Germany	Effects on muscles of WBV (Gallileo 2000) in combination with physical therapy for treating female stress urinary incontinence	5–30 Hz; oscillations with average cycle length 40 ms, 5 mm, 4 min	Physical Therapy	n = 29, crossover random design using three groups all receiving combinations of therapy in varying sequencing (PT and Gal, PT then Gal, Gal then PT), two training units of 30 min PT per week, and vibration training 2× 4 min, over 24 weeks with 12-week follow-up	WBV with PT improves subjective and objective parameters of stress urinary incontinence.

| Wakeling et al (2002), *J Appl Physiol*, 93:1093–1103 | Muscle activity damps the soft-tissue resonance that occurs in response to pulsed and continuous vibration | 10–65 Hz, 5 mm, a cycle of 3 s of vibration followed by 3 s of no platform movement. During each vibration period, the frequency and amplitude of the platform vibration were kept constant. Frequencies of 10.0, 13.1, 17.1, 22.3, 29.1, 38.1, 49.7 and 65.0 Hz were tested. These eight frequencies were presented in a randomized block. The randomized block was then repeated five times so that the subject experienced a total of 40 periods of vibration in each test | Standing on a vibrating platform with slight knee-flexion angle of 23° | $n = 20$, 10 male, 10 female | Elevated muscle activity and increased damping of vibration power occurred when the frequency of the input was close to the natural frequency of each soft tissue. Natural frequency of the soft tissues did not change in a manner that correlated with the frequency of the input. It is suggested that soft-tissue damping may be the mechanism by which resonance is minimized at heel strike during running. |

Table 6.3 Synopsis of research into WBV, compiled by Martin Krause and Alfio Albasini—cont'd

Researchers, names	Type of research	Dose	Exercise	Methodology	Outcome
Xie et al (2006), *Bone* 39:1059–1066	Low-level vibrations influence on bone resorption and formation	WBV 45 Hz (0.3g) for 15 min per day, and WBV with 10 s rest		8-week-old female mice, $n = 18$	3 weeks of WBV did not negatively influence body mass, bone length or chemical bone matrix properties of the tibia. Inhibition of bone resorption, site-specific attenuation of declining levels of bone formation, maintain a high level of matrix quality.
Yamazaki et al (2002), *Spinal J* 2:415–420	Vibratory loading decreases extracellular matrix and matrix metalloproteinase gene expression in rabbit annulus cells	2, 4, 6 and 8 hours of vibration loading, 0.1g, 6 Hz	Passive loading on annulus cells in vitro	Rabbit	Aggrecan, collagen type III, matrix metalloproteinase-3 expression was suppressed.

The Activities-specific Balance Confidence (ABC) Scale*

Instructions to Participants:

For each of the following, please indicate your level of confidence in doing the activity without losing your balance or becoming unsteady from choosing one of the percentage points on the scale form 0% to 100%. If you do not currently do the activity in question, try and imagine how confident you would be if you had to do the activity. If you normally use a walking aid to do the activity or hold onto someone, rate your confidence as you were using these supports. If you have any questions about answering any of these items, please ask the administrator.

The Activities-specific Balance Confidence (ABC) Scale*

For each of the following activities, please indicate your level of self-confidence by choosing a corresponding number from the following rating scale:

0%   10   20   30   40   50   60   70   80   90   100%
no confidence   completely confident

"How confident are you will not lose your balance or become unsteady when you...

1. ...walk around the house? ___%
2. ...walk up or down stairs? ___%
3. ...bend over and pick up a slipper from the front of a closet floor ___%
4. ...reach for a small can off a shelf at eye level? ___%
5. ...stand on your tiptoes and reach for something above your head? ___%
6. ...stand on a chair and reach for something? ___%
7. ...sweep the floor? ___%
8. ...walk outside the house to a car parked in the driveway? ___%
9. ...get into or out of the car? ___%
10. ...walk across a parking lot to the mall? ___%
11. ...walk up or down a ramp? ___%
12. ...walk in a crowded mall where people rapidly walk past you? ___%
13. ...are bumped into by people as you walk through the mall? ___%
14. ...step onto or off an escalator while you are holding onto a railing? ___%
15. ...step onto or off an escalator while holding onto parcels such that you cannot hold onto the railing? ___%
16. ...walk outside on icy sidewalks? ___%

* Powell, LE & Myers AM. The Activities-specific Balance Confidence (ABC) Scale. *J Gerontol Med Sci* 1995; 50(1): M28-34

Figure 6.8

TINETTI BALANCE ASSESSMENT TOOL

Tinetti ME, Williams TF, Mayewski R, Fall Risk Index for elderly patients based on number of chronic disablities. Am J Med 1986:80:429-434

PATIENTS NAME _____   D.o.b _____   Ward _____

BALANCE SECTION

Patient is seated in hard, armless chair;

			Date		
Sitting Balance	Leans or slides in chair	= 0			
	Steady, safe	= 1			
Rises from chair	Unable to without help	= 0			
	Able, uses arms to help	= 1			
	Able without use of arms	= 2			
Attempts to rise	Unable to without help	= 0			
	Able, requires >1 attempt	= 1			
	Able to rise, 1 attempt	= 2			
Immediate standing Balance (first 5 seconds)	Unsteady (staggers, moves feet, trunk sway)	= 0			
	Steady but uses walker or other support	= 1			
	Steady without walker or other support	= 2			
Standing balance	Unsteady	= 0			
	Steady but wide stance and uses support	= 1			
	Narrow stance without support	= 2			
Nudged	Begins to fall	= 0			
	Staggers, grabs, catches self	= 1			
	Steady	= 2			
Eyes closed	Unsteady	= 0			
	Steady	= 1			
Turning 360 degrees	Discontinuous steps	= 0			
	Continuous	= 1			
	Unsteady(grabs, staggers)	= 0			
	Steady	= 1			
Sitting down	Unsafe (misjudge distance, falls into chair)	= 0			
	Uses arms or not a smooth motion	= 1			
	Safe, smooth motion	= 2			
		Balance score		/16	/16

Figure 6.9

Berg Balance Scale

Description:
14-item scale designed to measure balance of the older adult in a clinical setting.

Equipment needed: Ruler, 2 standard chairs (one with the arm rests, one without)
Footstool or step, Stopwatch or wristwatch, 15 ft walkway

Completion:
>   **Time:**   15-20 minutes
>   **Scoring:**   A five-point ordinal scale, ranging from 0-4. "0" indicates the lowest level
>   of function and "4" the highest level of function. Total Score = 56

Interpretation: 41-56 = low fall risk
                        21- 40 = medium fall risk
                        0 - 20 = high fall risk

Criterion Validity:
"Authors support a cut off score of 45/56 for independent safe ambulation".

Riddle and Stratford, 1999, examined 45/56 cutoff validity and concluded:
- Sensitivity = 64% (Correctly predicts fallers)
- Specificity = 90% (Correctly predicts non-fallers)
- Riddle and Stratford encouraged a lower cut off score of 40/56 to assess fall risk

Comments: Potential ceiling effect with higher level patients. Scale does not include gait items

Norms:
Lusardi, M.M. (2004). Functional Performance in **Community Living Older Adults**.
Journal of Geriatric Physical Therapy, 26(3), 14-22.

Table 4. Berg Balance Scale Scores: Means, Standard Deviations, and Confidence Intervals by Age, Gender, and Use of Assistive Device

Age(y)	Group	N	Mean	SD	CI
60-69	Male	1	51.0	—	35.3 - 66.7
	Female	5	54.6	0.5	47.6 - 61.6
	Overall	6	54.0	1.5	52.4 - 55.6
70-79	Male	9	53.9	1.5	48.7 - 59.1
	Female	10	51.6	2.6	46.6 - 56.6
	Overall	19	52.7	2.4	51.5 - 53.8
80-89	Male	10	41.8	12.2	36.8 - 46.8
	Female	24	42.1	8.0	38.9 - 45.3
	No Device	24	46.3	4.2	44.1 - 48.5
	Device	10	31.7	10.0	28.3 - 35.1
	Overall	34	42.0	9.2	38.8 - 45.3
90-101	Male	2	40.0	1.4	28.9 - 51.1
	Female	15	36.9	9.7	32.8 - 40.9
	No Device	7	45	4.2	40.9 - 49.1
	Device	10	31.8	7.6	28.4 - 35.2
	Overall	17	37.2	9.1	32.5 - 41.9

Figure 6.10

Berg Balance Scale

Name: _____   Date: _____

Location: _____   Rater: _____

ITEM DESCRIPTION	SCORE (0-4)
Sitting to standing	_____
Standing unsupported	_____
Sitting unsupported	_____
Standing to sitting	_____
Transfers	_____
Standing with eyes closed	_____
Standing with feet together	_____
Reaching forward with outstretched arm	_____
Retrieving object from floor	_____
Turning to look behind	_____
Turning 360 degrees	_____
Placing alternate foot on stool	_____
Standing with one foot in front	_____
Standing on one foot	_____

Total   _____

GENERAL INSTRUCTIONS
Please document each task and/or give instructions as written. When scoring, please record the lowest response category that applies for each item.

In most items, the subject is asked to maintain a given position for a specific time. Progressively more points are deducted if:
- the time or distance requirements are not met
- the subject's performance warrants supervision
- the subject touches an external support or receives assistance from the examiner

Subject should understand that they must maintain their balance while attempting the tasks. The choices of which leg to stand on or how far to reach are left to the subject. Poor judgment will adversely influence the performance and the scoring.

Equipment required for testing is a stopwatch or watch with a second hand, and a ruler or other indicator of 2, 5, and 10 inches. Chairs used during testing should be a reasonable height. Either a step or a stool of average step height may be used for item # 12.

Figure 6.11

Berg Balance Scale

SITTING TO STANDING
INSTRUCTIONS: Please stand up. Try not to use your hand for support.
( ) 4   able to stand without using hands and stabilize independently
( ) 3   able to stand independently using hands
( ) 2   able to stand using hands after several tries
( ) 1   needs minimal aid to stand or stabilize
( ) 0   needs moderate or maximal assist to stand

STANDING UNSUPPORTED
INSTRUCTIONS: Please stand for two minutes without holding on.
( ) 4   able to stand safely for 2 minutes
( ) 3   able to stand 2 minutes with supervision
( ) 2   able to stand 30 seconds unsupported
( ) 1   needs several tries to stand 30 seconds unsupported
( ) 0   unable to stand 30 seconds unsupported

If a subject is able to stand 2 minutes unsupported, score full points for sitting unsupported. Proceed to item #4.

SITTING WITH BACK UNSUPPORTED BUT FEET SUPPORTED ON FLOOR OR ON A STOOL
INSTRUCTIONS: Please sit with arms folded for 2 minutes.
( ) 4   able to sit safely and securely for 2 minutes
( ) 3   able to sit 2 minutes under supervision
( ) 2   able to able to sit 30 seconds
( ) 1   able to sit 10 seconds
( ) 0   unable to sit without support 10 seconds

STANDING TO SITTING
INSTRUCTIONS: Please sit down.
( ) 4   sits safely with minimal use of hands
( ) 3   controls descent by using hands
( ) 2   uses back of legs against chair to control descent
( ) 1   sits independently but has uncontrolled descent
( ) 0   needs assist to sit

TRANSFERS
INSTRUCTIONS: Arrange chair(s) for pivot transfer. Ask subject to transfer one way toward a seat with armrests and one way toward a seat without armrests. You may use two chairs (one with and one without armrests) or a bed and a chair.
( ) 4   able to transfer safely with minor use of hands
( ) 3   able to transfer safely definite need of hands
( ) 2   able to transfer with verbal cuing and/or supervision
( ) 1   needs one person to assist
( ) 0   needs two people to assist or supervise to be safe

STANDING UNSUPPORTED WITH EYES CLOSED
INSTRUCTIONS: Please close your eyes and stand still for 10 seconds.
( ) 4   able to stand 10 seconds safely
( ) 3   able to stand 10 seconds with supervision
( ) 2   able to stand 3 seconds
( ) 1   unable to keep eyes closed 3 seconds but stays safely
( ) 0   needs help to keep from falling

STANDING UNSUPPORTED WITH FEET TOGETHER
INSTRUCTIONS: Place your feet together and stand without holding on.
( ) 4   able to place feet together independently and stand 1 minute safely
( ) 3   able to place feet together independently and stand 1 minute with supervision
( ) 2   able to place feet together independently but unable to hold for 30 seconds
( ) 1   needs help to attain position but able to stand 15 seconds feet together
( ) 0   needs help to attain position and unable to hold for 15 seconds

Figure 6.12

Berg Balance Scale continued......

REACHING FORWARD WITH OUTSTRETCHED ARM WHILE STANDING
INSTRUCTIONS: Lift arm to 90 degree. Stretch out your fingers and reach forward as far as you can. (Examiner places a rule at the end of fingertips when arm is at 90 degrees. Fingers should not touch the ruler while reaching forward. The recorded measure is the distance forward that the fingers reach while the subject is in the most forward lean position. When possible, ask subject to use both arms when reaching to avoid rotation of the trunk.)
( ) 4   can reach forward confidently 25 cm (10 inches)
( ) 3   can reach forward 12 cm (5 inches)
( ) 2   can reach forward 5 cm (2 inches)
( ) 1   reaches forward but needs supervision
( ) 0   loses balance while trying/requires external support

PICK UP OBJECT FROM THE FLOOR FROM A STANDING POSITION
INSTRUCTIONS: Pick up the shoe/slipper, which is place in front of your feet.
( ) 4   able to pick up slipper safely and easily
( ) 3   able to pick up slipper but needs supervision
( ) 2   unable to pick up but reaches 2-5 cm (1-2 inches) from slipper and keeps balance
independently
( ) 1   unable to pick up and needs supervision while trying
( ) 0   unable to try/needs assist to keep from losing balance or falling
TURNING TO LOOK BEHIND OVER LEFT AND RIGHT SHOULDERS WHILE STANDING
INSTRUCTIONS: Turn to look directly behind you over the left shoulder. Repeat to the right. Examiner may pick an object to look at directly behind the subject to encourage a better twist turn.
( ) 4   looks behind from both sides and weight shifts well
( ) 3   looks behind one side only other side less weight shift
( ) 2   turns sideways only but maintains balance
( ) 1   needs supervision when turning
( ) 0   needs assist to keep from losing balance or falling

TURN 360 DEGREES
INSTRUCTIONS: Turn completely around in a full circle. Pause. Then turn a full circle in the other direction.
( ) 4   able to turn 360 degrees safely in 4 seconds or less
( ) 3   able to turn 360 degrees safely one side only 4 seconds or less
( ) 2   able to turn 360 degrees safely but slowly
( ) 1   needs close supervision or verbal cuing
( ) 0   needs assistance while turning

PLACE ALTERNATE FOOT ON STEP OR STOOL WHILE STANDING UNSUPPORTED
INSTRUCTIONS: Place each foot alternately on the step/stool. Continue until each foot has touch the step/stool four times.
( ) 4   able to stand independently and safely and complete 8 steps in 20 seconds
( ) 3   able to stand independently and complete 8 steps in > 20 seconds
( ) 2   able to complete 4 steps without aid with supervision
( ) 1   able to complete > 2 steps needs minimal assist
( ) 0   needs assistance to keep from falling/unable to try

STANDING UNSUPPORTED ONE FOOT IN FRONT
INSTRUCTIONS: (DEMONSTRATE TO SUBJECT) Place one foot directly in front of the other. If you feel that you cannot place your foot directly in front, try to step far enough ahead that the heel of your forward foot is ahead of the toes of the other foot. (To score 3 points, the length of the step should exceed the length of the other foot and the width of the stance should approximate the subject's normal stride width.)
( ) 4   able to place foot tandem independently and hold 30 seconds
( ) 3   able to place foot ahead independently and hold 30 seconds
( ) 2   able to take small step independently and hold 30 seconds
( ) 1   needs help to step but can hold 15 seconds
( ) 0   loses balance while stepping or standing

STANDING ON ONE LEG
INSTRUCTIONS: Stand on one leg as long as you can without holding on.
( ) 4   able to lift leg independently and hold > 10 seconds
( ) 3   able to lift leg independently and hold 5-10 seconds
( ) 2   able to lift leg independently and hold ≥ 3 seconds
( ) 1   tries to lift leg unable to hold 3 seconds but remains standing independently.
( ) 0   unable to try of needs assist to prevent fall

(   ) **TOTAL SCORE (MAXIMUM = 56)**

Figure 6.12—cont'd

Guidelines for the Six-Minute Walk Test

The following elements should be present on the 6MWT worksheet and report:

Lap Counter: __ __ __ __ __   __ __ __ __ __   __ __ __ __ __

Patient name: _____   Patient ID# _____

Walk# __ _____   Tech ID: _____   Date: _____

Gender: M F   Age: ___   Race: ____ Height: ___ft __ ____in, _____meters

Weight: ____ ____ lbs, __ ____kg   Blood pressure: _____/ _____

Medications taken before the test (dose and time): _____

Supplemental oxygen during the test: No Yes, flow ___ ___ L/min, type _ _____

	Baseline	End of Test
Time	___:___	___:___
Heart Rate	____ __	__ _____
Dyspnea	__ ____	___ ___ (Borg CR10 Scale®)
Fatigue	____ __	___ ___ (Borg CR10 Scale®)
SpO$_2$	____ __ %	___ __%

Stopped or paused before 6 minutes?   No   Yes, reason: ____ _____ _____ ___

Other symptoms at end of exercise: angina   dizziness   hip, leg, or calf pain

Number of laps: __ __ (x 60 meters) + final partial lap: _____ __ meters =

Total distance walked in 6 minutes: _____ __ meters

Predicted distance: ___ ____ meters   Percent predicted: _____ __%

Tech comments:

Interpretation (including comparison with a preintervention 6MWD):

Figure 6.13 Guidelines for the Six-Minute Walk Test (*American Journal of Respiratory and Critical Care Medicine*, 166/111-117, American Thoracic Society (2002))

*The Borg CR10 Scale® (© Gunnar Borg)

0 Nothing at all
0.5 Very, very slight (just noticeable)
1 Very slight
2 Slight (light)
3 Moderate
4 Somewhat severe
5 Severe (heavy)
6
7 Very severe
8
9
10 Very, very severe (maximal)

Figure 6.13—cont'd This Borg scale should be printed on heavy paper (11 inches high and perhaps laminated) in 20-point type size. At the beginning of the 6-min exercise, show the scale to the patient and ask the patient: 'Please grade your level of shortness of breath using this scale.' Then ask: 'Please grade your level of fatigue using this scale.' At the end of the exercise, remind the patient of the breathing number that they chose before the exercise and ask the patient to grade their breathing level again. Then ask the patient to grade their level of fatigue, after reminding them of their grade before the exercise.

*For basic information about scale construction, metric properties, correct administration etc., it's necessary to read the book (Borg, G. 1998, *Borg's Perceived Exertion and Pain Scales*, Human Kinetics) and relevant folder.

Scales and Instructions can be obtained for a minor fee from Dr. G. Borg and his company, Borg Perception, Rädisvägen 124, 16573 Hässelby, Stockholm, Sweden. Phone: 46-8-271426 or E-mail: borgperception@telia.com.

Index

Notes: Page numbers suffixed with 'f' indicate figures: page numbers suffixed with 't' indicate tables.